MW01076865

WHAT WENT WRONG

WHAT WENT WRONG

America's Covid Response and Lessons for the Future

GREGORY E. PENCE

ROWMAN & LITTLEFIELD

Lanham • Boulder • New York • London

Rowman & Littlefield
Bloomsbury Publishing Inc, 1385 Broadway, New York, NY 10018, USA
Bloomsbury Publishing Plc, 50 Bedford Square, London, WC1B 3DP, UK
Bloomsbury Publishing Ireland, 29 Earlsfort Terrace, Dublin 2, D02 AY28, Ireland
www.rowman.com

British Library Cataloguing in Publication Information Available

Library of Congress Cataloging-in-Publication Data Available

ISBN 9781538199701 (cloth)
ISBN 9781538199725 (ebook)

For product safety related questions contact productsafety@bloomsbury.com.

∞™ The paper used in this publication meets the minimum requirements of American
National Standard for Information Sciences—Permanence of Paper for Printed Library
Materials, ANSI/NISO Z39.48-1992.

Contents

Contents

PREFACE

In October 2019, two months before Covid erupted in China, the Johns Hopkins Center for Health Security partnered with the *Economist* to run mock responses of 195 countries to dangerous pandemics.[1] The exercise spent millions of dollars, and thousands of experts worked hours running simulations. Its resulting "Global Health Security Index" lamented the unpreparedness of most countries, but America, it claimed, was best prepared.

That claim then may have seemed plausible. After all, America had many advanced medical centers, from Johns Hopkins to Stanford, to UCLA to my University of Alabama at Birmingham (UAB) Medical Center, where Jeanne Marrazzo, the person who later took over Anthony Fauci's job, chaired our department of infectious diseases.

On January 24, 2020, while briefing congresspeople about the outbreak in China, the director of the Centers for Disease Control and Prevention, Robert Redfield, told Congress: "We are prepared for this."[2]

Nothing could've been further from the truth.

The Hopkins Center and Redfield could have been thinking about America's impressive medical institutions, including the Centers for Disease Control and Prevention (CDC), the Health and Human Services (HHS) agency, the Food and Drug Administration (FDA), the National Institutes for Health (NIH), the vast network of veterans hospitals, and the agency that Anthony Fauci headed, the National Institute of Allergies and Infectious Diseases (NIAID). Ironically, we had even created the Office of National Security and Pandemic Preparedness.

We had the world's best pharmaceutical industry, allied with a mighty biotech industry, one that made everything from test tubes to artificial limbs to hemodialysis machines to ventilators, and critically, that could quickly create tests for new diseases and process thousands of new tests each day.

When faced in the past with lethal infectious diseases, America had sometimes performed well. When Ebola erupted in Guinea, Liberia, and Sierra Leone in March 2014, the Obama administration sent three thousand personnel from the CDC, the NIAID, and the Department of Defense, as well as seven thousand civilians.[3] Although eight thousand Africans died of the twenty-two thousand infected, the virus was contained by teaching proper burial techniques, supplying four hundred tons of personal protective equipment (PPE), and creating two hundred special burial sites.

America acted so effectively then that other countries modeled their responses on ours. Yet no country today would model its response on how we dealt with Covid-19 (henceforth just "Covid").

And given our own history with pandemics, we should've acted better. In the nineteenth century, we suffered three waves of cholera. In 1918–1920, we weathered the Spanish flu.[4] In the 1950s, polio terrified American parents as it left kids paralyzed, so we funded Jonas Salk's vaccine with the March of Dimes. In the twentieth century, we experienced swine flus and annual rounds of seasonal flu, developing quadrivalent vaccines each year. In 1998, we had experienced SARS-COV-1 (henceforth, SARS1).

Yet somehow, when Covid came knocking, our famous can-do attitude went missing; instead of answering the call, something went terribly wrong. As Lawrence Wright wrote in *The Plague Year* (2021):

> *Into this turbulent, deeply troubled, but prideful society, the coronavirus would act as a hurricane of change, flattening the*

most powerful economy in the world, leveling not the physical cities but the idea of cities, strewing misfortune and blame and regrets along the tens, the hundreds, the thousands, and hundreds of thousands of obituaries. No country would escape the destruction the virus inflicted, but none had as much to lose as America.[5]

As the BBC showed long lines in February 2020 of Italian trucks carrying Covid dead to cemeteries, a skeptical parent from rural Alabama asked me, "Do you really think Covid will come here?" A century before, as cholera broke out in India and crept through the Middle East, then slipped into Montreal and later down into New York, Alabamians had asked similar questions, and of course, the answer had always been not "if," but "when."

Alas, during Covid in America, the attitude of "we're all in this together" got lost in political-cultural battles. Instead of banding together to fight a dangerous germ, we battled each other.

We battled over facts; we battled over who had authority; we battled over who could be trusted. Everyone became a bioethicist as everyone opined about who should be vaccinated first, or if at all. Social epistemology, a new, cutting-edge field in philosophy, loomed large as people debated which news media could be trusted, a problem that continues today.

And isn't it amazing that America has had no official inquiry about Covid, despite America having the third-highest per capita Covid death rate in the world (3,300 per million people)?[6] Moreover, given America's relatively small population (compared to India or Indonesia), why did it suffer three hundred thousand more deaths than any other country?[7]

An official inquiry almost happened, as physician-bioethicist Ezekiel Emanuel wrote in 2022: "We were supposed to lay the groundwork for a National Covid Commission. The Covid Crisis

Group formed at the beginning of 2021, one year into the pandemic. We thought the U.S. government would soon create or facilitate a commission to study the biggest global crisis so far in the twenty-first century. It has not."[8] That commission never survived a divided Congress, so Emanuel's task-force members published their views unofficially.[9]

In contrast, Britain began an official inquiry in December 2023, one that will continue until 2026, asking whether it could have handled Covid better (its death toll was among the worst of the European countries) and focusing on the administration of Boris Johnson.[10]

This stuff matters. We're talking during the pandemic about lots of deaths, including *unexplained* deaths. As Anthony Fauci concluded, 1.1 million deaths for the richest country in the world, one with some of the world's best medical facilities, is "unacceptable."[11] And importantly for this book, Covid's official death count only partly explains what went wrong. Worldwide, the United Nations judged that Covid officially killed seven million but estimates that the world also suffered thirty-three million "excess" deaths.[12]

Between 2020 and 2024 in America, at least 401,000 excess deaths occurred.[13] A crucial ethical question concerns whether those more than four hundred thousand Americans needed to die. Might some of those deaths have been prevented? How many were caused not just by Covid, *but by America's response to Covid?*

Americans already suffer from Covid amnesia, shuffling all the bad things into an epistemic black hole, just as we did after the Great Flu of 1919.

There will be facts about Covid documented by medical historians, but the narratives will be set long before the histories appear. In the meantime, our polarized American culture tells people divergent stories about Covid.

The American past offers a lesson here. After the Civil War, Confederate generals and Southern newspaper editors began the saga of the Lost Cause, the view that brave, honorable Confederate soldiers fought not over slavery, but over states' rights and to repel attacks of "Northern Aggression." The Daughters of the Confederacy erected monuments in Southern cities to Robert E. Lee and Stonewall Jackson, and they curated children's textbooks to downplay slavery and exalt noble soldiers defending the freedom of Southerners.[14]

The North extolled a different view, at first portraying soldiers as fighting to keep the country together and later as opposing slavery. Gradually, the identity of Northerners faded into being just Americans, but that did not happen in the South, where a distrust of Washington's Yankees lingered for centuries. It did not help that many Southerners descended from Scottish, Irish, and German ancestors who had been persecuted by centralized, authoritarian governments.

It is helpful to recall, too, the work about how memory is shaped by Elizabeth Loftis and Ulric Neisser, who proved that memory was not a simple, objective reception of facts, but a subjective, dynamic process greatly influenced by people's motivations, expectations, and experiences. After the space shuttle *Challenger* blew up, Professor Neisser asked a large class to write down how they felt when they heard the news. Years later, he asked them how sure they were about what they had written years before. Everyone was very sure, but upon opening their previous statement, half admitted their memory was erroneous.[15]

Loftis, often called as a defense witness about the reliability of memories of eyewitness accounts of crimes, proved that memory was not an immutable recording of objective reality, but something reconstructed and pliable, especially shapeable by what people around a person said about the event. For example, few people in New York City personally saw the Twin Towers go down, but many saw them do so on television. After a while, especially as New Yorkers embellished stories to make themselves eyewitnesses, they came to believe they saw what they didn't.[16]

I review these studies about the pliability of memory because already I hear people saying, "I had Covid four times, and it was nothing," or "Half the people I knew died of Covid." People who had colds, flus, or infections may later reconstruct those events as Covid. People who suffer chronic conditions such as tinnitus, muscular fatigue, or lasting immune problems may claim all were caused by Covid.

The battle lines are being laid down: either by progressives or conservatives, each having views about Long Covid, the origins of Covid, the cost of lockdowns, and who led best. Even the major newspaper and cable news networks take sides, too, such that the other side rarely gets a fair shake.

So, here we are, four years after Covid started, with various authors attempting to spin views of what went wrong. Some make Anthony Fauci an heroic official suffering under a crazy president, whereas others make Fauci the personification of an arrogant Washington insider who was out of touch with the ordinary American businessman.

In this book, I try to impartially investigate how America handled Covid, the results of which could help us do better the next time, either with a bird flu or with a new SARS-COV-3. The book also raises some crucial questions about how the media and politicians on both sides suppressed unpopular views. But being impartial is hard, because many forces now attempt to shape how the pandemic is viewed.

Not everyone will like my answers. Both conservatives and liberals made mistakes handling Covid, big mistakes. In writing this book, I have tried to follow the evidence, even as it sometimes made me change the positions with which I began.

The overall message of this book is that balancing different values in fighting pandemics is not just a medical decision, but a much more general one of public policy. Fighting disease and death is one value, but preventing business failures, preventing overdose deaths, and preventing years of loss of learning in kids are other values. Choosing the right trade-offs among these values is not a medical decision, but a complex ethical one, one for which doctors and medical officials have no special wisdom.

Finally, issues in this book pertain not only to handling future pandemics, but also to the safety of xenotransplants, where the possibility exists of mutant coronaviruses arising inside such transplants and creating new pandemics, a threat that, I believe, has been unappreciated by the public.

NOTES

1. Michael Lewis, *The Premonition: A Pandemic Story*, Norton, 2021, xii.

2. Lawrence Wright, "The Plague Year," *New Yorker*, January 4 and 11, 2021, 23.

3. The White House, "The Administration's Response to Ebola," National Archives, March 15, 2015, https://obamawhitehouse.archives.gov/ebola-response#:~:text=Since%20the%20start%20of%20the,person%20U.S. %2Dbacked%20civilian%20response.

4. Joshua Loomis, *Epidemics: The Impact of Germs and their Power over Humanity*, New York: Prager, 202.

5. Wright, 18–19.

6. David Wallace-Wells, "Interview with Anthony Fauci," *New York Times Magazine*, April 30, 2023, 39. Wallace-Well's reference for the per-capita figure is from *Our World in Data*, which reports 3,300 Covid deaths per million for the United States, 3,280 for the United Kingdom, and so on. Peru had 6,400 Covid deaths per million, but this is not a country that America normally compares its health statistics against.

7. John Elflein, "Coronavirus (COVID-19) in the U.S.—Statistics & Facts," *Statista*, December 18, 2023.

8. The Covid Crisis Group, *Lessons from the Covid War: An Investigative Report*, Public Affairs Press, 2023, 1.

9. The Covid Crisis Group, *Lessons from the Covid War: An Investigative Report*, Public Affairs Press, 2023.

10. Mark Landler, "Johnson Defends Covid Response but Apologizes for Victims' Pain," *New York Times*, December 3, 2023.

11. Wallace-Wells, 39.

12. "The Pandemic's True Death Toll," *Economist*, January 20, 2024.

13. John P. A. Ioannidis et al., "Variability in excess deaths across countries with different vulnerability during 2020–2023," *Proceedings of the National Academy of Sciences*, November 29, 2023, https://www.pnas.org/doi/10.1073/pnas.2309557120.

14. An excellent account of the conflicting narratives that people constructed about the American Civil War is by Caroline Janney, *Remembering the Civil War: Reunion and the Limits of Reconciliation*, The University of North Carolina Press, 2013.

15. Ulric Neisser and R. Fivush, *The Remembering Self: Construction and Accuracy in the Self-Narrative*, Cambridge: Cambridge University Press, 2008.

16. Rachel Avis, "How Elizabeth Loftis Changed the Meaning of Memory," *New Yorker*, March 29, 2021.

The Prime Directive

Having been a bioethicist for nearly fifty years in a medical center, having taught medical students for over thirty years, having served on committees with physicians, having taught graduate courses in UAB's School of Public Health, and having served on our Institutional Review Board for twenty-two years, I understand how medical professionals reflexively respond to pandemics: *stop infections and save lives.* Their response is so deep that it's automatic and unquestioned. I call this response "the Prime Directive."

Unthinking, uncontested acceptance of the Prime Directive explains some of what went wrong during Covid in America. It explains why lockdowns continued too long, why many restaurants and small businesses failed, why lockdowns poured gasoline on America's polarized politics, why many doctors and nurses quit, and why many teachers and first responders did the same.

In the cultural battles that plagued America during Covid, the Prime Directive represented arrogant elites in the Northeast dictating values to Americans who lived in "flyover land." Yet those Americans there had their lives upended by the Prime Directive and had little say about its adoption or implementation.

Of course, the Prime Directive had intellectual heft. In ethics, it implicitly invoked a Rawlsian theory of justice: a just society first protects its most vulnerable people. John Rawls, the late Harvard political philosopher, argued this way in his *A Theory of Justice* (1971), specifically, that under a veil of ignorance in a social contract, self-interested citizens would vote to structure a just society first to build a safety net for its most vulnerable citizens.

But where Rawls's theory itself is vulnerable was in defining "the most vulnerable." The Prime Directive defines them as "most likely to die from Covid," but others might define them as "most likely to die from postponing surgery," "most likely to commit suicide," or even "most likely to be unable to read because of lockdowns."

Other scholars noticed how the Prime Directive became dominant during Covid. Didier Fassin, a medical anthropologist in the School of Social Science at the Institute for Advanced Study in Princeton, enumerated the many great sacrifices and harms imposed by lockdowns during Covid and concluded that, "Such sacrifices had only one *raison d'être*: the reduction of mortality due to the coronavirus. They were deemed the price required to save lives."[1]

In March 2020, as Americans watched what was happening in China and around the world, the Prime Directive made sense. Everyone then had so many questions: How deadly was Covid? How infectious was its virus? If you were infected, how likely were you to die? In early 2020, no one knew the answers.

As we struggled through 2020 and then endured 2021, some things started to become clear. We started to learn that lockdowns unintentionally harmed people, especially poor people, especially parents who had to leave unsupervised kids at home. In retrospect, I fear that few professionals like me, who could work from home, and who never had a paycheck in doubt, never fully appreciated the toll this took on people who, for example, were trying to keep open a small bakery and who had put their life's savings into such a business.

AN ALTERNATIVE: FOCUSED PROTECTION

James T. Reason, a psychology professor at the University of Manchester, around 1990 proposed a "Swiss Cheese Model" of accident prevention, arguing that the likelihood of accidents in industrial production or aviation could be drastically reduced by creating layers of protection, each of which might not be perfect, but which together produced a high level of safety.[2]

In early 2020, Ian McKay, an Australian virologist, built on Reason's model and produced an infographic illustrating how it could be employed during the Covid pandemic.[3] In this defense, which went viral, McKay suggested that masks must not only be worn by everyone, but they also must be worn correctly, frequently washed, and have multiple layers of cloth woven tightly. Another "slice of cheese" was physical distancing, which McKay said was the most effective preventive measure that could be taken.[4]

Countries that used this "Swiss Cheese Defense" limited travel across their borders; provided safe places for infected people to quarantine; supported salaries while people quarantined; circulated fresh air in buildings; and created clear, transparent, evidence-based messages.

Rather than lockdowns, Reason's and McKay's Swiss Cheese Defense urged reducing capacity to 20 percent at gyms, bars, restaurants, and stores, allowing many such businesses to limp along, but also stopping viral spread in large gatherings.[5] Such "capacity limits" worked best in towns with a low incidence rate of the virus.

In March 2020, three professors advanced the Swiss Cheese Defense as a possible strategy to fight Covid. They called it "Focused Protection." They were Sunetra Gupta, a professor of infectious diseases at the University of Oxford; Jay Bhattacharya, an MD/PhD professor of the economics of health care at Stanford University; and Martin Kulldorff, a biostatistician and professor of medicine at Harvard University, who had also served on the FDA's drug and vaccine safety committees.

Focused Protection argued that lockdowns, especially ones lasting years, harmed people too much and overemphasized preventing death and hospitalization while ignoring the harms of suicide, overdose deaths, domestic abuse, and business failures. They argued that restrictions of freedom should match risks to specific groups. One-size-fits-all restrictions needlessly harmed too many people who didn't need protection.

Scientifically, they argued that leaders should follow the evidence about who needed restrictions and about who needed special protections. Importantly, Focused Protection posited that vulnerable people required special protection. Frail clients in nursing homes must be carefully protected, as well as residents of "congregate living facilities" such as homeless shelters and prisons.

For example, if it turned out that Icelanders, with their unique and somewhat-homogenous genetic inheritance, only got mild sniffles from SARS2 and never needed hospitalization, then it would be absurd to close in-person teaching at Icelandic schools, shut down gymnasiums and restaurants, and lock down Icelandic society to prevent mass cases of a runny nose.

On the other hand, consider the harms of loss of work. Lockdowns created massive unemployment for the twenty-one million Americans who filed for benefits during Covid. Many others experienced "under employment,"[6] working gig jobs such as driving for Uber or making deliveries of food and supplies.

While it's true that trillions of new dollars in federal aid helped workers limp through Covid, unemployment can profoundly affect self-esteem. For some workers, the loss of a job can create depression and anxiety, especially when employers later rehired younger workers. Moreover, for millions in the United States, medical coverage depended on employment, so the loss of employment resulted in the loss of medical coverage or resorting to the Medicaid benefits used by the poor.

Lockdowns during Covid created many angry owners of restaurants and bars. My favorite, James Beard Award–winning restaurant in Birmingham never reopened after lockdowns forced its closure in 2020, and many others only reopened with half the hours and the staff of pre-Covid days.

Eric Klingenberg's book *2020: One City, Seven People, and the Year Everything Changed* documented seven New Yorkers' experiences with Covid that first year, among them Daniel Presti, who had poured his life's savings into opening Mace's Public House in a residential part of Staten Island in late November 2019.[7] When Covid hit New York City, Governor Andrew Cuomo ordered all bars and restaurants closed on March 14. Presti initially accepted the lockdown and tried to survive with takeout orders, but over the next year, things changed for Mr. Presti.

As Governor Cuomo fought Mayor deBlasio and both fought President Trump, and as messages from Anthony Fauci changed and contradicted themselves, Presti went from being apolitical to being an anti-government activist. By October of 2020, Mace's Public House had permanently closed, and Presti had become an ardent critic of lockdowns and the government's response to Covid.

How many Daniel Prestis did extended lockdowns create? How many failed businesses have blamed contradictory and confusing mandates from public health and politicians?

United States citizens were unaccustomed to massive government regulation of their lives, so they resisted control. Protests erupted in Germany, Holland, and Italy over lockdowns, led by owners of small businesses. In Canada, truck drivers led huge protests, even shutting down Ottawa for a week in protest of mandatory vaccinations directed by Justin Trudeau.[8]

Besides business failures, Focused Protection lamented the increased deaths from addiction and alcoholism that the lockdowns created. Because millions of people seeking recovery could not meet face-to-face, because national resources were diverted to fighting Covid, and because medical personnel understandably were more focused on Covid, the needs of addicted people went unmet. Isolated and without work, it was easy for too many to turn to alcohol and drugs.

Before Covid and for years, you could not open a newspaper or watch the news without reading a story about the opioid epidemic and related deaths. At the start of the pandemic, opiate overdoses killed about seventy thousand American each year, a figure that had risen alarmingly from forty-five thousand in 2015.

Suddenly, Covid bumped all these stories into oblivion. For three years, the media could not write about anything but Covid. Meanwhile, in the background, that "other epidemic" worsened, as we left behind our former rate of overdose deaths of seventy thousand a year. By January 2021, the number had jumped to ninety-five thousand, and by 2022, to 108,000; then by January 2023, to 110,000.[9]

After the Sackler family and Purdue Pharma flooded America with OxyContin, existing pills got laced with cheap fentanyl. In both cases, political infighting and Covid distracted everyone so much that *no one noticed that a decade of overdose deaths would soon kill more Americans than Covid.* In Baltimore alone, in the six years between 2018 to 2024, six thousand people died of overdoses.[10]

When a parent died of an overdose, few people noticed the children left behind, yet between 2011 and 2021, over 321,000 American children lost a parent to a drug overdose.[11] Tragically, American Indian, or Alaska Native, families had the highest rate of overdoses, which tragically left thousands of orphans behind.

Deaths from alcoholism also soared. According to the CDC, during our Covid years, an additional forty thousand Americans died from alcoholism—from 138,000 a year in 2019 to 178,000 in each year of 2020 and 2021.[12] As Covid cleared the highways, police patrolled them less, but reckless and drunk driving soared, and with it, deaths from drunk drivers. Before Covid, drunk drivers killed about ten thousand Americans a year, but in each year of 2021 and 2022, they killed 13,500.[13]

Domestic violence also increased. Being at home all day, sometimes with hyperactive young children, can fray anyone's nerves. Add alcohol and drugs to the mix, on top of preexisting tensions in a family, and violence can and often does erupt against partners, against children, against the elderly, and even against pets, who during lockdowns were also increasingly abandoned.[14]

Less-noticed damage also occurred during lockdowns to people with disabilities. Special-needs kids need extra human contact, which is intensive and expensive and which withers away during lockdowns. Seniors in nursing homes also wither without social contact, and they fared miserably locked in their rooms with just a television and a computer screen. Millions of post-surgery patients and those who suffer from muscular diseases need daily physical therapy, which became impossible to obtain during lockdowns. And for every person who was actually homeless or hungry, ten more worried constantly about a similar fate.

Postponed medical care also created extra, non-Covid deaths during lockdowns. Fearing exposure to Covid in medical clinics, cancer patients postponed or stopped chemotherapy; very few organ transplants occurred during the first year of Covid. People even feared calling 911 for heart attacks or going to emergency rooms when having strokes, worried that the ER was already overwhelmed or that they would catch Covid there.

Another casualty of fear of going to emergency rooms during Covid in America concerned pregnancy-related deaths. In 2019, about seven hundred American women suffered such a death, but in 2021, in the middle of the pandemic, that figure jumped by 500 to over 1,200—so an additional 500 pregnant women may have died needlessly, an appalling number.[15]

Although it is difficult to know the exact number of excess deaths that were caused by the Covid lockdowns, the numbers are surely high. As mentioned, while the official worldwide count is seven million Covid deaths (as of January 2024),[16] excess deaths were at least 33.5 million.[17] These worldwide figures are stunning, especially because they suggest that *more* people died because of responses to Covid than from Covid itself. As the *Economist* concluded in early 2024, "These data make clear that Covid-19 has led to the deaths of far more people than official statistics suggest."[18]

Although the review of the numbers here can be numbing, remember that each death statistic represents a life lost. At the very least, we need to know what our pandemic policy cost in *American* lives.

We know that "officially," as of March 2024, 1,161,000 Americans died of Covid (more later, on how "Covid deaths" are "officially" defined).[19] But how many excess deaths occurred between 2020 and 2023? How many Americans would have normally died during those four years, how many officially died of Covid, and how many were excess deaths?

According to a report from the National Academy of Sciences in 2024, the number of non-Covid, excess deaths was one hundred thousand a year—or four hundred thousand excess dead Americans for 2020–2024.[20] It states, "The United States of America is a striking case, with extremely high cumulative excess death rates despite high per capita GDP."

In contrast, Sweden, which largely pursued Focused Protection, had an extremely low rate of non-Covid excess deaths. The report added, "Canada, United Kingdom, the United States of America, and Chile had very poor performance specifically among the nonelderly, while Slovenia, France, and Poland showed the opposite pattern."[21]

THE SUPPRESSION OF FOCUSED PROTECTION

The three professors who publicized Focused Protection originally met at a think tank in the small town of Great Barrington in western Massachusetts in the fall of 2020 and drafted a statement about Focused Protection as a strategy for managing Covid. Unfortunately, the think tank in Great Barrington, a libertarian one opposed to regulations to reduce global warming, puffed up their statement to title it as the pompous "Great Barrington Declaration.[22] A better phrase would have been "Focused Harm Reduction" or some similar phrase using that term *harm reduction*. Henceforth, I shall just call it "Focused Protection."

As the Covid pandemic wore on, some experts agreed with the Great Barrington Declaration and started to dissent from the Prime Directive, emphasizing that it might be doing more harm than good, especially to young children and poorer families. San Francisco infectious disease doctor Monica Gandhi, who came to Covid with decades' worth of experience treating HIV/AIDS patients, embraced the idea and called it "harm reduction applied to Covid."[23] Along with the above three professors, as the pandemic progressed, Gandhi questioned whether closing schools really helped children (the topic of a later chapter).

Physician and medical historian Howard Markle joined Gandhi's critique. Markle had spent his lifetime studying the history of medicine and pandemics. Early in 2020, he criticized China's draconian lockdowns, arguing that the incremental measures of Focused Protection could work as well or better.[24]

What happened next explains one thing that went wrong during Covid: leading authorities in public health quashed a reasonable alternative to managing the pandemic, that is, they suppressed all discussion of Focused Protection. After the Great Barrington Declaration, NIH director Francis Collins and Anthony Fauci actively encouraged doctors and scientists not to engage with the authors of this Declaration over evidence, but rather try to cancel them. Collins shamefully wrote that, "There needs to be a quick and devastating published take-down of its premises."[25]

In the *Washington Post*, Collins declared that Focused Protection wasn't science, but was dangerous. Fauci said that Bhattacharya and Kulldorff were like people in the 1980s who denied that HIV caused AIDS, terrible accusation coming from someone who had been a hero in the AIDS years. Yet in Great Britain by the fall of 2020, over 6,700 professionals had signed a petition supporting Focused Protection, and so it was never—as some critics claimed—just an idea of three "fringe" professors.[26]

The initial intolerance of Collins and Fauci is one of the saddest tales about "what went wrong" during Covid. When these two attacked champions of Focused Protection as political ideologues, the medical associations piled on.

Not only were such attacks philosophically intolerant, but they were also heavily class-based, because many professionals could do their jobs efficiently from their homes during lockdowns, but many people in lower-paying jobs could not. However, the most damaging criticism is that Collins and Fauci took the high moral ground that they were "following the science," when, in fact, they did not do so about Focused Protection.

Many forces suppressed Focused Protection. First, for obvious reasons, it clashed with the Prime Directive: keeping everyone employed might result in slightly higher "official" deaths from Covid. Second, American political discourse in the mass media typically then suffered from an "us versus them," black-or-white, attitude, with no nuanced middle. Behind such extreme political discourse was Donald Trump and his philosophical allies such as Ron DeSantis, who embraced Focused Protection as an alternative to lockdowns, but for the many professionals opposed to Trump, no good idea could be associated with him or DeSantis.

Finally, champions of Focused Protection were not leaders in public health—not in charge at the FDA, the CDC, or the NIH, and they were not insiders in Washington, DC. Leaders in public health such as Anthony Fauci claimed advocates should have vetted their ideas first with them, although their receptiveness to such ideas is in doubt.

Still, it is difficult to understand why the authors of this Great Barrington Declaration never got a fair shake by American public health officials, or the media aligned with them (MSNBC, CNN, the *New York Times*, *USA Today*, and the *Washington Post*). Critics seized on one statement—that "herd immunity" was ultimately their goal—and ignored the other tenets. Only the *Wall Street Journal*, sympathetic to businesses trying to survive the lockdowns, featured guest columnists sympathetic to Focused Protection.

Even more astonishing to both Libertarians and Europeans, MSNBC, CNN, the *New York Times*, *USA Today*, and the *Washington Post* seemed perfectly fine with the federal government drastically limiting civil liberties without any checks or balances, such as the right to assemble for religious services, even in cars in parking lots. As will be discussed later, this was the perfect opportunity for Donald Trump to declare a Public Health Emergency and expand the president's powers over both states and citizens. Why he didn't do so is still a mystery.

A typical takedown of Focused Protection was to attack the straw man, that its champions wanted no restraints on behavior and wanted many people quickly infected in order to obtain herd immunity. But *both sides* had the goal of obtaining herd immunity. The contentious point concerned whether years-long lockdowns had to continue—with all their consequent harms—to achieve that goal, or whether some less-drastic approach might work better.

Four years after the first reports emerged of a new virus in Wuhan, China, evidence had mounted about the horrific harm of lockdowns, and in late 2023 Francis Collins tried to limit the damage to his reputation. It is worth quoting him here because he comes to understand the criticism of Focused Protection about the harms of lockdowns and that the "public health mindset" was "another mistake we made":

> *If you're a public-health person and you're trying to make a decision, you have this very narrow view of what the right decision is, and that is something that will save a life. So, you attach infinite value to stopping the disease and saving a life. You attach zero value to whether this actually totally disrupts people's lives, ruins the economy, and has many kids kept out of school in a way that they never quite recovered.*[27]

Only four years later did Francis Collins acknowledge that the Great Barrington Declaration "could have been a great opportunity for a broad scientific discussion about the pros and cons" of Focused Protection, but he fails to admit his mistake in actively trying to cancel the authors and to stop discussion of its ideas. This is like saying that protests about the Vietnam War could have been a great opportunity in the political community for discussing the merits of that war, but not admitting that you previously and strenuously tried to prevent all the protestors from gathering to protest.

FOCUSED PROTECTION IN AMERICA

San Francisco. Focused Protection accidentally worked in America in some surprising places, "accidentally" because it was never officially endorsed in these places as official policy. In San Francisco, which had been the epicenter of AIDS deaths in the 1980s and which afterward became a national model of long-term care for HIV-infected adults, an existing infrastructure helped reduce Covid deaths, as well as hard-earned trust in local officials in public health.

Unlike most cities, where nursing homes are private, or even private and run to maximize profits, San Francisco's Department of Public Health owned Laguna Honda, a facility that housed

750 residents, and that department of public health did a full-court press to keep its residents safe. As Joe Nocera and Bethany McLean conclude in the *The Big Fail*:

> *The San Francisco experience should cause us to reflect on the Great Barrington Declaration. Its primary message was that the most important thing to do in a pandemic is protect the most vulnerable. That's what San Francisco did. . . . It's more than a little ironic that the city with the least tolerance for pandemic dissent would end up following the path put forth by the dissidents' most vilified document.*[28]

New York versus Florida. After talking with the authors of the Great Barrington Declaration, Florida's governor Ron DeSantis adopted Focused Protection. He protected the vulnerable elderly in nursing homes, but otherwise ordered few restrictions.

Contrast that with what happened in New York. On March 2, 2020, an Orthodox Jewish congregation north of New York City experienced a cluster of cases. Governor Andrew Cuomo instituted an aggressive containment zone around New Rochelle. Unknown to Cuomo, a thousand other New Yorkers were already infected, undoubtedly because New York City's huge subway, bus, and train systems—supporting nearly four billion rides each year and with rush hours making people stand close together—was a massive amplification system.

By April, America had two hundred thousand cases, eighty-four thousand in New York—with one thousand American deaths in one day.[29] Ambulances bringing sick Covid patients to emergency rooms howled through New York City's five boroughs, causing massive anxiety. To house expected overflows, the Army Corps of Engineers built a field hospital in the Javits Convention Center, and the USNS *Comfort* docked in New York City's harbor. Many Covid patients required intensive care and ventilators, which became scarce, and bioethicists debated how to distribute them.

Governor Cuomo held daily press briefings, pleading for a national response and for help, which antagonized President Trump, who was focused on keeping businesses and schools open.

The most powerful evidence that DeSantis had adopted the best strategy with Focused Protection came two years after Covid began. Consider that the states of New York and Florida had roughly the same populations: 19.8 million New Yorkers versus 21.7 million residents in Florida. Yet after four years of the pandemic, New York had 6,500,000 cases of Covid and 77,325 Covid deaths; Florida had 7,350,000 cases and 84,176 Covid deaths.

At the end of 2022, "New York State led the nation in population loss," according to *Newsday*, a Long Island newspaper, while "Florida leads US population growth for the first time in 65 years," said *Bloomberg News*. Between 2020 and 2022, New York State lost two million people, and Florida gained two million.

Of course, Florida had no income tax, and New York had a big one. Florida had no mass transit system running across its major city. On the other hand, Florida had more senior citizens per capita, and as consequence, more nursing homes.

Nursing Homes

New York's governor failed to protect nursing homes and under-reported the deaths there, whereas Florida's governor protected its nursing home residents more. This is both understandable and a big deal.

If you're pursuing lockdowns as your primary weapon against a pandemic, then nothing special needs to be done for nursing homes because *everything* falls under the same rules of social distancing, masking, and super cleansing. On the other hand, if you're pursuing Focused Protection, then you will focus on the people whom Covid will most likely kill, namely, those over the age of eighty with several medical problems.

If someone is very fit at eighty, they may be the functional equivalent of sixty and hence, not live in a nursing home. On the other hand, someone might have so many medical problems at age sixty that functionally they're the medical equivalent of eighty. When you visit nursing homes, you understand this because some people there look to be in their eighties but are in their sixties. Thus, it makes sense to vaccinate those in nursing homes first, to protect them the most, and to hire extra, vaccinated staff to serve them.

Finally, if someone in such a home gets Covid and needs to go to a hospital, if that person is successfully treated, they should only be returned to the nursing home if they are 100 percent not infectious. It appears that some nursing homes in New York were forced to accept former patients infected with Covid back from hospitals too early and subsequently infected everyone there. Governor Cuomo tried to disguise this mistake, leading to an investigation.[30]

FOCUSED PROTECTION WORLDWIDE
Niger
Consider the Republic of Niger, a landlocked African nation, perhaps the world's poorest country, which also contains its youngest citizens, with a median age of fifteen. Half its citizens are under the age of twenty, with 75 percent under thirty.[31] Of Niger's twenty-seven million people in 2023, only 1.5 million were over the age of sixty.

Niger's youth made Focused Protection its best option. During the Covid pandemic, if you wanted to produce the greatest number of life years for the greatest number of people, Focused Protection for Niger was not only permissible, but morally required.

By October 25, 2020, Niger officially had only 1,200 SARS2 infections and sixty-nine Covid deaths. Lockdown would have harmed twenty million young citizens, merely to protect fewer-than-seventy citizens from potentially dying from Covid? Would lockdowns have even worked in such a poor country? Although some infections and deaths in Niger surely went unreported, according to WHO, it had less than ten thousand infections and three hundred deaths.[32]

China

The cost of pursuing zero Covid infections in China with lockdowns now seems too high. China's economy, which had previously been growing at 5 percent each year, drastically shrank. A billion Chinese suffered tight controls about where they could work, eat, walk, or travel. If one person in an apartment complex tested positive, everyone in the complex had to leave for quarantine camps for three to four weeks, or the complex was sealed off from the world.

Things worsened so much in China that at a Foxconn plant, where iPhones were made, workers started committing suicide, and after a bad fire there, mass protests started against Covid restrictions. When Chinese citizens saw ordinary people unmasked next to each other in the stands at the FIFA World Cup matches, more protests erupted. The fans demanded to know how Chinese restrictions could still be justified when soccer fans elsewhere could sit in huge crowds watching the games. Fearing its dwindling economy, in late 2022 China abruptly canceled all internal controls.

Sweden

Sweden adopted Focused Protection and fared well. Seeing itself as a relatively healthy country with medical care for all, it decided that a softer approach might work best, although at first, champions of the Prime Directive ridiculed its approach.

Citizens around the world in lockdowns saw pictures of Swedes in bathing suits in 2021 crowded together on wharfs and beaches, an eerie, open-air experiment. Restaurants and bars remained mostly open throughout the whole pandemic. Because Sweden didn't shut down its economy, many Americans began to admire Sweden's approach and wonder why the same approach wouldn't work in the United States.

Critics said that Sweden's approach sacrificed fragile senior citizens. Rather than sacrificing their grandparents to the virus, Swedish officials countered that they were saving Swedes from suicide, increased addiction, domestic violence, and poverty.

Sweden had some justification for its approach. With its comprehensive medical system giving free medical care to all citizens, Swedes did not fear losing medical coverage through a job loss, nor were high co-payments a worry for the sick. As one Scandinavian said, "You're not as concerned about catching the virus, because you know that, if you do, the state is paying for your health care."[33]

In December 2020, as its hospitals struggled to handle many sick patients, and stung by criticism that it wasn't doing enough for the elderly in its nursing homes, Sweden temporarily banned gatherings of more than eight people and implemented some restrictions on travel. But by and large, Sweden kept open K–12 schools and colleges, as well as businesses and its overall economy.

By 2024, things looked much better for how Sweden had handled Covid.[34] Its rate of excess deaths was low, far below Australia or New Zealand.[35] Its mean age of death from Covid was eighty-two.[36] It also had a high rate of vaccination among its citizens, a sign of trust in government and public health.

America's National Academy of Sciences concluded in Sweden's favor, stating that if America had followed Sweden's policies, as many as 1,600,000 non-Covid, excess deaths could have been prevented.[37] Moreover, and most importantly, as we'll see in the next chapter, Sweden barely closed its schools, and its children emerged from the pandemic with normal progression in reading and math ability.[38]

CONCLUSIONS

Public health allied with medicine and hospitals in fighting disease and tried to save lives. Its axiology or value priorities did not include educating kids, but rather, keeping them safe. The same was true for businesses and restaurants: public health's job was to keep them free of Covid, not to help them prosper.

Just as it's bad to have "one ring to rule them all," so it's bad in public policy for one value to rule them all. No matter if it's saving lives of seniors, fighting global warming, or preserving mental health, every aspect of life involves conflicting values and trade-offs.[39]

Although we often heard that we should "follow the science," the science during Covid was shifting, uncertain, and hard to know. In such circumstances, many values and stakeholders compete against each other, and truth to tell, *leaders in public health have no special moral expertise in deciding which trade-offs are best for everyone.*

That is a hard lesson for the many schools of public health to accept. Nevertheless, managing pandemics can't just involve the Prime Directive, because many other stakeholders also have interests that count. Think of a large university, with schools of public health, nursing, and medicine, but also with schools of business, engineering, and agriculture, all with students and alumni who have different needs during a pandemic.

What we also saw during Covid was a surprising asymmetry between the plans conceived beforehand and what really happened. Focused Protection should have been more sympathetically discussed. Had it been, fewer overall excess deaths in America would have occurred; fewer restaurants, gyms, and small businesses would have failed; and America would not have needed to borrow trillions from the next generation to keep its economy going (more on this in a later chapter).

Unfortunately, champions of the Prime Directive lumped advocates for Focused Protection with anti-vaxxers, and the federal government's chief agencies collaborated with major social media companies to repress posts from both groups, as will also be discussed later.[40]

NOTES

1. Didier Fassin and Marion Fourcade, *Pandemic Exposures: Economy and Society in the Time of the Coronavirus*, HAU Books, 2022, Society for Ethnographic Theory, www.haubooks.org.

2. James T. Reason, *Human Error*, Cambridge: Cambridge University Press, 1990; James Reason, "The Contribution of Latent Human Failures to the Breakdown of Complex Systems," *Philosophical Transactions of the Royal Society of London. Series B, Biological Sciences*, April 14, 1990, 327 (1241): 475–84.

3. Siobhan Roberts, "Beating the Pandemic with a Swiss Cheese Defense," *New York Times*, December 7, 2020.

4. Carmine Gallo, "The Virologist Who Created a 'Swiss Cheese' Metaphor to Explain the Pandemic Has a Message for Educators," *Forbes*, December 10, 2020, https://www.forbes.com/sites/carminegallo/2020/12/10/the-virologist-who-created-a-swiss-cheese-metaphor-to-explain-the-pandemic-has-a-message-for-educators/?sh=28ca3cd36335.

5. Yaryna Serkez, "A 20 Percent Shutdown Could Be Enough," *New York Times*, December 17, 2020, A23.

6. Eric Klinenberg, *2020: One City, Seven People, and the Year That Changed Everything*, Knopf, 2024.

7. Ibid.

8. "Ottawa's state of emergency quell protests against vaccine mandates?" *Economist*, February 7, 2022.

9. CDC, National Center for Health Statistics, "Provisional Drug Overdose Death Counts," March 13, 2024, https://www.cdc.gov/nchs/nvss/vsrr/drug-overdose-data.htm.

10. Alissa Zhu, Nick Thieme, and Jessica Gallagher, "Almost 6,000 Dead in 6 Years: How Baltimore Became the U.S. Overdose Capital," *New York Times*, May 23, 2024, A1.

11. Ken Alltucker, "A startling number of kids lost parents to overdoses. Experts on how to buck the trend," *USA TODAY*, May 10, 2024, A1.

12. CDC, "Deaths from Excessive Alcohol Use in the United States," February 24, 2024, https://www.cdc.gov/alcohol/features/excessive-alcohol -deaths.html.

13. Scott Calvert, "Drunk-Driving Deaths Up, Arrests Fall," *Wall Street Journal*, May 3, 2024, A3.

14. M. L. Evans et al., "A Pandemic within a Pandemic: Intimate Partner Violence during COVID-19," *New England Journal of Medicine*, December 10, 2020, 383:24, 2303–4.

15. Mike Stobbe, "U.S. pregnancy deaths dropped in 2022, after COVID spike," *STAT*, March 16, 2023.

16. World Health Organization, "WHO COVID-19 Dashboard," https://data.who.int/dashboards/COVID19/deaths?n=c.

17. "The Pandemic's True Death Toll," *Economist*, January 20, 2024.

18. Ibid.

19. CDC, COVID Data Tracker, accessed March 5, 2024, https://covid .cdc.gov/covid-data-tracker/#datatracker-home.

20. John P. A. Ioannidis et al., "Variability in excess deaths across countries with different vulnerability during 2020–2023," *Proceedings of the National Academy of Sciences*, November 29, 2023, https://www.pnas.org/doi /10.1073/pnas.2309557120.

21. Ibid.

22. "Great Barrington Declaration," https://gbdeclaration.org/.

23. Monica Gandhi, *Endemic: A Post-Pandemic Playbook*, Mayo Clinic Press, 2023, 6.

24. Howard Markel, "Will the Largest Quarantine in History Just Make Things Worse?" *New York Times*, January 27, 2020.

25. Editorial, "How Fauci and Collins Shut Down the COVID Debate," *Wall Street Journal*, December 21, 2021.

26. "COVID-19: Group of UK and US experts argues for 'focused protection' instead of lockdowns," *British Medical Journal*, October 7, 2020, 371.

27. Francis Collins, quoted in *Wall Street Journal*, December 30–31, 2023, A12.

28. Joe Nocera and Bethany McLean, *The Big Fail: What the Pandemic Revealed about Who America Protects and Who It Leaves Behind*, Penguin 2023, 257–58.

29. Khrysgiana Pineda, "Reviewing Thousands of Deaths, Millions of Cases," *USA Today*, July 24, 2020, A4.

30. Jesse McKinley and Luis Ferré-Sadurní, "New Allegations of Cover-Up by Cuomo over Nursing Home Virus Toll," *New York Times*, February 21, 2021; Brendan J. Lyons, "FBI, U.S. attorney in Brooklyn probing Cuomo administration on nursing homes," February 17, 2021,

Times Union; "Andrew Cuomo Faces House Subpoena over COVID Deaths in Nursing Homes," *New York Times*, March 5, 2024.

31. World Health Organization, "Coronavirus Disease: Niger."

32. Ibid.

33. Thomas Harr, quoted by Peter Goodman, "Sweden Has Become the World's Cautionary Tale," *New York Times*, July 7, 2020, updated July 15, 2020.

34. Brain Polumbo, "More Data Vindicate Sweden's Hands-Off Pandemic Approach," *Washington Examiner*, April 4, 2023.

35. Insändare, "Obefogad kritik från Coronakommissionen," February 28, 2022.

36. "Veckorapport om COVID-19, vecka 18" (PDF). Folkhälsomyndigheten, May 8, 2020.

37. John P. A. Ioannidis et al., "Variability in excess deaths across countries with different vulnerability during 2020–2023," *Proceedings of the National Academy of Sciences*, November 29, 2023, https://www.pnas.org/doi/10.1073/pnas.2309557120.

38. A. E. Hallin et al., "No Learning Loss in Sweden during the Pandemic: Evidence from Primary School Reading Assignments," *International Journal of Educational Research* 114 (2022): 102011; doi:10.1016/j.ijer.2022.102011.

39. On how fighting global warming exclusively can harm other values, see Bjorn Lomborg, "'Follow the Science' Leads to Ruin," *Wall Street Journal*, March 14, 2024, A15.

40. Bret Swanson, "COVID Censorship Proved to Be Deadly," *Wall Street Journal*, July 7, 2023; Jenin Younes and Aaron Kheriaty, "The White House Censorship Machine," *Wall Street Journal*, January 9, 2023, A17; Allysia Finley, "Public Distrust of Health Officials Is Fauci's Legacy," *Wall Street Journal*, January 9, 2023, A17.

A Brief Overview of Viruses, Pandemics, and Covid

Even though most people know about Covid and its virus, SARS COV-2 (henceforth, just "SARS2"), it will be helpful to review some facts about it for ideas that appear in the following chapters.

VIRAL EPIDEMICS BEFORE COVID

Germs that spread infectious diseases to humans fall into three types: bacteria, protozoa, and viruses. Bacteria cause tuberculosis, syphilis, bubonic plague, and typhus. Protozoa cause diseases such as malaria and African sleeping sickness.

Viruses cause smallpox, yellow fever, HIV/AIDS, polio, and forms of influenza, including the Great Flu of 1918. Bacteria, much larger than viruses, could be seen with early microscopes created around 1600, but viruses are so tiny that it wasn't until 1930 that electron microscopes allowed scientists to visualize them.

A virus' capacity to damage its host is its *virulence*, and its ability to spread is its R_0 *value* (pronounced "R naught"). A person infected with SARS2 infects on average 2 to 2.5 new people. In other words, its R_0 value is 2–2.5; most seasonal flus have an R_0 value of 1.3.

Immunity from the virulence of viruses comes in degrees and in several kinds: *vaccinated immunity* gives immunity to death and serious illness, which is what Covid vaccines conferred; *natural immunity*, which occurs after recovering from infection with Covid; and *sterilizing immunity*, which is the complete ability to prevent infection.

Only sterilizing immunity guarantees against first infection or reinfection. Some people mistakenly believed that Covid vaccines gave sterilizing immunity and were surprised when vaccinated people became reinfected or infected others. They then mistakenly inferred that all vaccines were worthless.

Herd immunity, an ambiguous phrase, has the central idea that not every member needs to be vaccinated for the entire herd to be protected. In most developed countries by 2024, enough people had endured Covid or were vaccinated that herd immunity had been achieved. Among other things, this means that the *community spread* of Covid had stopped occurring from person to person. "Herd immunity" is ambiguous because it could mean the herd is immune from death, from serious disease, from mild disease, or even from infection altogether.

HISTORICAL VIRAL PANDEMICS

Pandemics caused by viruses are not new, and lessons can be learned from past mistakes in handling them. The so-called Spanish flu of 1918, which originated in Kansas, swiftly killed between fifty and one hundred million people worldwide. Some cities acted correctly, but others, such as Philadelphia, encouraged officials to be deceitful about the virus' lethality. Philadelphia infamously allowed its Liberty Loan Parade to sell war bonds, creating an amplification system for the virus. In early 1918, 150,000 citizens there were infected, and 17,500 died, one of the worst rates of infection and death in the world.[1]

This flu virus entered Philadelphia from sailors, who were allowed to disembark from their ships and carouse in downtown bars. Some Philadelphians blamed them and their loose morals, an historical pattern called *blaming the victim*, or *scapegoating*, which dates to the bubonic plague in the fourteenth century (the "Black Death"), when traveling Jews were blamed (when, in fact, fleas carried by rats spread the germ).

In this century, the *Proceedings of the National Academy of Sciences* identified two key factors of cities that successfully contained this virus: (1) When the first cases appeared, they quickly banned large gatherings, instituted temporary lockdowns, enforced the wearing of masks and social distancing, and (2) they did not reverse these actions quickly.[2] In addition, successful cities issued consistent, evidence-based, non-politicized messages about efforts to control the virus.

Even a century ago, scientists knew that wearing masks slowed the spread of germs. What many did not learn during Covid was that wearing a mask not only reduced the chances of others getting infected, but also, upon exposure, wearing a mask reduced the chances of serious illness for the person wearing it, i.e., "the more virus you get into your system, the more likely you are to get sick."[3]

Pandemics create great fear, which can create the need to blame some group. Sometimes *purification rituals* accompany blame, in which society attempts to clean itself of culprits, and where history's worst example is human sacrifice.

Viruses transmitted smallpox and yellow fever, both of which have caused historical pandemics. The first effective vaccine developed was for smallpox, which had killed millions of natives of the Americas, who lacked the acquired immunity of Europeans. The virus of yellow fever most likely originated in Africa in the 1600s, and eventually most Africans inherited immunity to it, but in contrast to smallpox, many Europeans had no inherited immunity to yellow fever and easily died from it.

In the twentieth century, the polio virus frightened many Americans, especially in 1952, when sixty thousand children became mysteriously infected and three thousand died. Others were left paralyzed, doomed to live their entire lives in iron lungs. Eventually, scientists learned that fecal matter in water carried the virus, and by 1955, Jonas Salk had created an effective polio vaccine.

The world also suffered from the HIV virus that causes AIDS. The simian version of HIV had lived in remote parts of Africa for centuries, and although it occasionally infected a human, isolation and difficulty traveling kept it from infecting many other humans.

By 1980, however, interstates, airplanes, and large cities in Africa allowed it to spread far more quickly, creating a crisis in 1981, when it infected blood supplies and when infected people had unprotected sex and shared needles.

HIV created great fear, and gay men with multiple partners, as well as IV-drug users, were blamed for spreading it. Initially, public health officials in America and France lied about the safety of the blood supply from HIV infection (a pattern Chinese officials may still be doing today), leading to many needless infections and skepticism about whether such officials could be trusted. During the 1980s, Anthony Fauci became a target of AIDS activists, who wished for faster trials for antiretroviral drugs, which—to his everlasting credit—Fauci eventually facilitated.

SARS-COV-1 (SARS1)

In the spring of 2003, the coronavirus named SARS-COV-1 originated in China in Asian palm civets (vaguely catlike, small mammals), leapt to cave-dwelling horseshoe bats in the southwest province of Yunnan, and then jumped to humans.[4] The bat-to-human interaction is important because it may have occurred again with SARS2, and it certainly will occur again.

SARS1 caused severe acute respiratory syndrome (SARS). Coronaviruses exist on a spectrum and include the viruses causing common colds. Many nonhuman animals experience coronaviruses and carry them, especially bats and pigs.

Airplanes helped SARS1 travel to Hong Kong and Toronto. One Canadian infected 257 Torontonians. Infections there from an orthopedic ward spread to another 361 Canadians. Panic ensued, and thousands of Torontonians voluntarily quarantined in their homes. For a few months, Canadians feared interacting with Asians, who were blamed for the virus.

Singapore's government quickly identified eight thousand citizens who had been exposed to the virus and forced them into quarantine. Singapore compensated them for lost income from missed workdays, which Canada did not, resulting in widespread noncompliance in Canada.

Although most who caught SARS1 survived, many afterward had long-term problems, including shortness of breath, chronic lung disease, and kidney problems. Even three years after the outbreak in Toronto, many survivors experienced musculoskeletal pain and fatigue, like chronic fatigue syndrome, now called myalgic encephalomyelitis, or ME/CFS.[5] These sequelae predicted that some people infected with SARS2 would experience similar long-term problems, which is today called Long Covid.

Although SARS1 infected less than nine thousand people worldwide, it still killed a thousand people. Why it disappeared is little understood, which became important for SARS2, because Donald Trump hoped that it, too, would disappear.

THE ASIAN FLU (1957) AND HONG KONG FLU (1968) PANDEMICS

Before SARS1 hit Asia and Canada in 2003, other viral epidemics had occurred, giving experience to leaders in countries on the Pacific Rim about how to respond. The Asian flu began in 1957 in Southeast Asia and killed two million people. For decades before, no one had seen such a deadly flu, so its emergence shocked the world, just as Covid did, and like SARS2, the Asian flu spread rapidly across the globe.

Later, in 1968, the Hong Kong flu followed a similar pattern, and although less deadly, it proved that flu could be a mass killer. This flu got its name because that July, a half million citizens of Hong Kong were suddenly sickened with flulike symptoms and swamped its hospitals.

Scientists at its flu center quickly identified the virus and alerted the WHO that a dangerous new virus had arrived. The virus soon spread to Vietnam during its war there with America, and American veterans carried it to Hawaii and then to San Diego. Eventually, it killed a million people worldwide, including a hundred thousand Americans.

Viruses causing seasonal flus each year kill twenty thousand to sixty thousand Americans, mostly elderly people with other medical problems. The first vaccine for seasonal flus came in 1936. Scientists today have identified several strains of flu, with A and B kinds and sub-kinds such as A/H1N1. The typical yearly vaccine tries to protect against four different strains—so-called quadrivalent vaccines. Because variations of the flu are always emerging, new vaccines are always needed.

In 2009, a deadly virus crossed over from pigs, a common pattern, but like the Spanish flu of 1918, it mainly killed young people. Scientists quickly created a vaccine for this "swine flu," and President Obama took an early dose in front of television cameras.

Many other viruses cause problems in humans, among them the Middle Eastern respiratory virus (thought to cross over from camels); the Zika virus, causing microcephaly in babies; hepatitis viruses (B, C, D, and E); West Nile virus; Norwalk virus, human papillomavirus virus (HPV); and herpesviruses.

A virus transmitted by mosquitoes causes dengue hemorrhagic fever, commonly called "breakbone fever" for the pain it causes in muscles and joints. Vaccines against dengue figure prominently in a later chapter, and this virus today causes a massive number of infections in Brazil, Venezuela, and Bangladesh, creating a great need to make safer, more effective vaccines against it.[6]

All viruses develop through a process called *antigenic drift.* It is important for understanding viruses and pandemics to realize that when viruses replicate, they are unstable and prone to errors. As microbiologist and pandemic historian Joshua Loomis explains,

> *Every time influenza viruses invade new cells and begin to replicate, the new genomes that are made contain small mutations. This is important because it increases the chances that a brand-new and deadly strain will emerge and ravage the population. This process by which influenza viruses mutate gradually . . . [is] antigenic drift. It is . . . why we must be inoculated with the flu vaccine annually: the flu strain present during one flu season may mutate enough the following year . . . that our immune system no longer . . . recognizes it.*[7]

In one case, antigenic drift from the H3N2 variant of influenza created the Hong Kong flu virus. Antigenic drift also illustrates evolution. Because antigenic drift constantly creates mutations in unstable viruses, new viruses always compete for survival with existing ones. A new virus that is more infectious than existing ones can reproduce faster and gain more successors.

However, a new virus can't be too lethal and kill its new hosts too fast, or else the hosts won't live long enough to infect new hosts. For example, the Ebola virus probably lived for centuries among bats in remote caves in Africa. Occasionally a person might have visited such a cave and gotten infected, but Ebola kills its hosts so fast that the victim never made it back to his home before he died, or if he did make it back there, everyone there died quickly, before they could travel elsewhere. Only when infected patient Charles Monet was flown in 1976 to a hospital in faraway

Nairobi did Ebola break out of rural Africa and become a threat to the world.[8]

Besides antigenic drift, another important concept to understand about viruses and pandemics is the *cytokine storm*. Cytokine storms may explain a mystery involving the Great Flu of 1918. Strangely, this virus severely sickened and killed mainly those under the age forty. Why? An old theory hypothesized that seniors had previously been exposed to flus and had acquired immunity to future flus—but then decades had passed without a similar flu, making 1918's young people "flu virgins."

A newer theory is that the Spanish flu killed the young by causing *cytokine storms*, where their younger, more fit immune systems overreacted to the virus, creating extreme inflammation and throwing everything at the virus, even to the point of destroying their own organs.

SARS-COV-2 (SARS2)

The coronavirus SARS-COV-2 (SARS2) originated in Wuhan, China. How it originated is still controversial, the subject of chapter 5.

Once SARS2 enters humans, it hijacks their cells, as if to say, "Don't do your usual job. Your job is now to help me multiply and help me make more virus."[9] Typically entering through the mouth and sinus passages, SARS2 "crawls progressively down the bronchial tubes" to enter the lungs, where it inflames mucous membranes, often damaging lung sacs and making it more difficult for the lungs to deliver oxygen to circulating blood.[10] From the lungs, the virus may enter the GI tract and other organs.

Primarily, this virus attacks the lungs, scarring them deeply and creating a medical condition called "acute respiratory distress syndrome" (ARDS). The sickest patients require ventilators, and if ventilators fail, a device known as ECMO (discussed in chapter 4).

Importantly, at some point, the coronavirus can enter the brain and central nervous system, causing the loss of taste and smell. Studies reveal that the virus may linger in the brains and central nervous systems of some infected patients for years.

THE CLINICAL COURSE OF COVID

The classic list of symptoms of initial infection with SARS2 includes the loss of sense of taste and smell, fever, chills, and anything that involves the lungs, such as a dry cough or shortness of breath. As physicians learned more, the list of symptoms expanded to include muscle aches, headaches, GI upset, diarrhea, muscular pain, swollen testes, and skin rashes. In rare cases, unusual rashes have appeared on fingers and toes, dubbed "Covid toes."[11]

About 80 percent of infected people have mild symptoms. Infected children may have no symptoms at all. The other 20 percent of infected adults experience serious flulike illness. In the United States, the SARS2 virus killed about 2 percent of those infected. It was especially lethal to those over the age of eighty with underlying medical problems. As a lung disease, it was especially dangerous for cigarette and marijuana smokers and vapers.[12] It killed men over fifty much more than women over fifty, although infected women were more likely to become Long Haulers.[13]

The antiviral drug remdesivir, at first given intravenously and then as an inhaled spray, offered some help.[14] Today, monoclonal antibodies, such as those made by Regeneron, and what was given to President Trump when he got Covid, block viral replication and seem to help.

Early in the pandemic, physicians put very sick patients on ventilators, sometimes even splitting one ventilator among two patients, but today they try to prevent this, using ventilators only as a last resort. Because some patients on ventilators stay in the hospital for weeks or several months, the toll on their organs and minds can be intense, such that full recovery may take many months or even years, leaving some with permanent "brain fog."[15]

Physicians eventually realized that too many Covid patients had been put on ventilators too soon, resulting in the scarcity of such machines, rationing, and demands for countries to manufacture more. Over time, physicians intervened aggressively to avoid ventilators, using steroids, supplemental oxygen, and proning—turning patients frequently so they can breathe more easily with damaged lungs.[16] Nevertheless, as discussed in chapter 4, surges of infection forced difficult decisions on many hospitals about who would receive breathing machines, especially surgically intense machines called ECMO (Extra-Corporeal Membrane Oxygenation).

Because the coronavirus is so infectious, hospital staff treating patients wore personal protective equipment (PPE) gear resembling space suits. This also meant that family members could not touch or visit sick relatives. Heart-wrenching scenes on television showed relatives outside nursing homes waving to despondent seniors inside.

Within twelve months, astute scientists and physicians realized that Covid mainly killed people over the age of eighty who suffered from several medical problems, such as chronic obstructive pulmonary disease, morbid obesity, cardiomyopathy, and diabetes. Using the standard distinction between chronological and functional age, Covid mainly killed patients who were functionally over the age of eighty.

Stating this fact is not blaming these victims. No one knows when lethal viruses may erupt and strike medically vulnerable patients. Moreover, all of us, if we live long enough, will become medically vulnerable.

NOTES

1. John Barry, *The Great Influenza: The Story of the Greatest Pandemic in History* (2004), Penguin, 2018.

2. *Proceedings of the National Academy of Sciences USA*, 104, no. 18 (2007): 7582–87.

3. Monica Gandhi, interviewed by Ailsa Chang on National Public Radio, July 20, 2020, "Growing Body of Evidence Suggests Masks Protect Those Wearing Them, Too."

4. Robin McKie, *The Guardian*, December 10, 2017.

5. Mayo Clinic, "Myalgic encephalomyelitis/chronic fatigue syndrome (ME/CFS)," https://mayoclinic.org/diseases-conditions/chronic-fatigue/symptoms-causes/sys-20360490.

6. "Dengue fever is surging in Latin America," *Economist*, April 25, 2024.

7. Loomis, 198.

8. Richard Preston, *The Hot Zone: The Terrifying True Story of the Origins of the Ebola Virus*.

9. William Shaffner of Vanderbilt University, quoted by Pam Belluck in "What Exactly Does This Virus Do in the Body?" *New York Times*, March 17, 2020, D7.

10. Ibid.

11. Steven Reinberg, "More symptoms of coronavirus: COVID toes, skin rashes," *Medical Press*, May 4, 2020.

12. Jan Hoffman, "Smokers and Vapers May Be at Greater Risk of Getting Coronavirus," *New York Times*, April 9, 2020.

13. CDC, "COVID-19 Mortality Update, 2022," May 5, 2023.

14. Katherine Wu, "Trial to Start on Version of Treatment One Inhales," *New York Times*, June 22, 2020.

15. Ed Yong, "COVID Can Last for Several Months," *Atlantic*, June 15, 2020.

16. "Proning COVID Patients Reduces Need for Ventilator," *Columbia University Medical Center News*, July 2, 2020.

Education Harms: Lockdowns vs. Focused Protection

Scientific evidence grew fastest during 2020 about children and their education. Doctors in large hospitals quickly learned that eighty-year-olds with multiple medical problems easily died from Covid, but not young kids, not high school students, and not college students. As one chart from the CDC explained, the likelihood of death from a Covid infection for an eighty-five-year-old exceeded that of a fourteen-year-old three hundred times.[1]

Monica Gandhi, the San Francisco doctor who ran HIV clinics for decades, complained that keeping schools closed for too long harmed children. Was this a big deal? Yes, especially for parents concerned about the fate of their kids. Between March 2020 and June 2021, at least sixty-two million children in American public-school systems didn't attend school in person; states such as California and Oregon kept their schools closed even longer.

Most private schools initially closed but quickly resumed in-person teaching. Consequently, the effect of lockdowns on children in private schools was minimal; it was much worse for children in public schools.

Internationally, from a study commissioned by the *Lancet* medical journal, 1.5 billion children worldwide in 195 counties were suddenly forced to learn remotely, with deleterious effects, especially on girls, who experienced greater depression, anxiety, and bullying than boys.[2]

By February 2020, Dr. Gandhi realized that SARS2 spared almost all children from serious illness.[3] She worried about damages to children's education from stopping in-person instruction, as well as damage to needy patients from postponed medical care, as well as damage to families from needless isolation, especially for elderly grandparents left alone.[4]

Children were also harmed in less-obvious ways. Reports of child abuse at home, usually first noticed by teachers in schools, dramatically dropped during Covid years.[5] Screenings for myopia and obesity stopped. Visits to ERs because of attempted suicides in teens soared, symptomatic of vastly increased incidence of mental health problems in kids.[6]

Dr. Gandhi claims that mainstream media focused too much on lockdowns and "did not effectively cover the damage from these ineffectual interventions, only in late 2022 did the media finally begin calling school closures a failed policy in that they caused harm to children without saving lives."[7]

When I think about it now, I realize I knew from the start that she was right: images on television from China and northern Italy showed elderly people coming to emergency departments, in ICU beds, and dying. I never saw a young child portrayed then as sick or dying.

When my grandnieces got infected, at ages five and eight, they ran around gleefully shouting, "I got Covid! I got Covid," delighted that they could stay home from school for two weeks. They were hardly sick, and when their parents, who were marathon runners, became infected, they had nothing worse than a mild flu.

At UAB, where I teach, and in my neighborhood in 2020 and 2021, dozens of kids in K–12 grades, and dozens more of my college students, became infected, but none of them became sick enough to visit an ER, much less be hospitalized, much less die. At UAB, some students and faculty got Covid and had to isolate.

In retrospect, after a few months, and certainly by the end of 2021, it became clear that children and adolescents fared no worse than having the flu for a few days.

What happened in closed, inner-city schools was worse: Many poor parents still had to work driving buses or stocking goods in stores, and with childcare facilities closed, many children had to stay at home with laptops, at best supervised by an older child. In such circumstances, many kids gave up: If they didn't know how to use the laptop, or if it didn't work, they had little help. In cities such as Baltimore, the absentee rate soared.

As Gandhi writes, "The United States (unlike the United Kingdom and European countries) failed to take into account the disease's profound age gradient when making recommendations for the public and schools, which led to polarization and discord in our response."[8]

Many good things happen when kids attend schools: their parents can work and feel their kids are safe; their kids may get the one good, nutritious meal of their day; problems of mental health or abuse can be detected; by interacting with other kids and teachers, kids learn social skills and develop character; in physical education classes, they exercise and learn different kinds of sports.

Amazingly, it is not clear that making kids wear masks reduced their risks of Covid infection. Of about six hundred observations and twenty-two more seemingly objective studies, almost all had strong biases toward masking, and in the end, a look-back analysis in 2023 concluded that "Real-world effectiveness of child mask mandates against SARS2 transmission or infection has not been demonstrated with high-quality evidence. The current body of scientific data does not support masking children for protection against Covid."[9]

Given the enormous harm of keeping kids in masks, keeping them six feet apart when in schools, closing daycare and nursery schools, and closing K–12 schools, it is scary how the slight danger to kids of Covid infection kept everything shuttered.

Joe Nocera and Bethany McLean, in *The Big Fail*, summarize the minimal dangers of Covid to kids in schools thus:

> *By midsummer 2020, when cities were trying to decide whether to reopen their public schools, 146,000 Americans had died of Covid-19. Exactly sixteen of them were children between the ages of five and fourteen.* More schoolchildren died from mass shootings.[10]

Nocera and McLean think state officials kept schools closed for three reasons. First, Americans had become phobic about the coronavirus and had stopped thinking rationally about chances of infection or death. (The author remembers taking packages that had been delivered to his house outside in the sun and wiping them down with Clorox wipes before opening them.)

Second, and important to understanding the continuing breakdown of trust in America, Trump wanted to reopen schools as quickly as possible. Given the lies, omissions, and outright deceptions that Trump pushed about Covid, journalists and officials suspected his motives. It didn't help that Florida governor Ron DeSantis also wanted schools open. CNN, MSNBC, and the *New York Times* could not second any proposal from him.

Third, Nocera and McLean emphasize that teachers themselves feared Covid. Some were elderly with medical problems. Bad enough to think about Sandy Hook, Uvalde, and other mass shootings in schools, but risking your life for Covid? In most American cities, teachers were Democrats, and three-quarters of them in urban systems paid dues in unions that had backed Joe Biden. The unions were focused on keeping teachers safe, distrusted Trump/DeSantis, and opposed reopening schools.

In this regard, they were like Europeans who championed the precautionary principle about innovations in biotechnology for genetically enhanced crops. According to this principle, you must prove in advance that the change won't create anything bad, an impossible task.

As mentioned, kids in private schools did not fall behind like kids in public schools. As one colleague told me about the private school in Michigan his kids attended:

They had mats for kids outside in big tents with heaters and kids spaced six feet apart. The outdoor air was a natural ventilation system. They never closed. The teachers never missed a paycheck. It was expensive but the school was amazing. It also brought all the parents together to support the school as never before.

And it wasn't just in America that educational disparities worsened by class. In September 2023, UNESCO declared that remote education had caused "staggering" inequalities worldwide in education and that overreliance on technology "worsened disparities and learning loss for hundreds of millions of students around the world, including Kenya, Brazil, Britain, and the United States."[11]

Half a billion students worldwide lacked internet connections. Because of bad internet connections or faulty hardware, one-third of K–12 students in America and Pakistan were "cut off from education." The promises of tech giants in Silicon Valley that digital tools would save and revolutionize education turned out to be mostly hollow.

A similar report by the U.S. Department of Education found that half of American students were a full year behind in at least one subject.[12] In many cases, students began 2022 at the same level as when they had started a year before.

David Nabarro, the WHO's special envoy for Covid-19, emphasized that "lockdowns have one consequence that you must never, ever belittle, and that is making poor people an awful lot poorer."[13]

As physician and vaccinologist Paul Offit concluded, "At first, the only strategy for decreasing Covid was to limit human-to-human contact. We closed businesses and shuttered schools. No one paid a bigger price for this approach than children, who suffered severely from lack of education and socialization. The effects of these deficits will no doubt be felt for years to come."[14]

During the first year of Covid, some closures of schools might have been justified, especially because it took a while to establish that kids were generally safe, but over time, what had begun as liberal solidarity with public health and against Trump became written in stone, such that anyone who suggested that keeping kids at home harmed them was blasted.[15]

By the end of 2022, evidence from many different studies started to accumulate showing that students in schools in the poorest areas fell behind much more than students in schools in middle-class areas, and that remote learning was inflicted on the former kind of student much longer than the latter, with the result that such students had lost almost half a year in math and half a year in reading. Moreover, back in school, they were much slower to make up for lost skills.[16]

Brown University researcher Emily Oster also found in her studies that school districts with Black and Hispanic students had less in-person teaching than those with mostly white students.[17] Oster warned very early during the pandemic, in the fall of 2020, in her article "Schools Aren't Super-Spreaders" in The *Atlantic*, that in-person teaching in schools was not an amplification system for SARS2.[18] Teachers and public health officials had given too much weight to how cold viruses spread, but SARS2 differed.

However, predetermined biases seemed to determine how any data were interpreted. In a study published in the *New England Journal of Medicine* about what happened when various school districts in Massachusetts lifted requirements to mask in school, the researchers found that lifting such mandates resulted in only forty-five new cases in students and staff per one thousand students. Amazingly, they then concluded that "Our results support universal masking as an important strategy for reducing Covid-19 incidence in schools."[19]

Importantly, the researchers do not distinguish between how many of the extra forty-five cases were among students and how many were among staff, but the important fact missing is that Covid infections among K–12 kids were generally not that serious. They did remark that extra cases mainly happened when the incidence of Covid was high in the surrounding community. But the researchers seemed to accept the Prime Directive: that the only goal was preventing infection.

In the fall of 2020, Governor Ron DeSantis kept Florida schools open, for which most national media portrayed him as a brutal Neanderthal. In retrospect, he led well on this issue.

Two years after her 2020 article in The *Atlantic*, Professor Oster published, "Let's Declare a Pandemic Amnesty," where she wrote, "There is an emerging (if not universal) consensus that schools in the US were closed for too long: The health risks of in-school spread were relatively low, whereas the costs to students' well-being and educational progress were high."[20]

By late 2023, even the editorial board of the *New York Times* agreed with the editorial board of the *Wall Street Journal*, concluding with the startling conclusion that "the school closings that took 50 million children out of the classroom at the start of the pandemic may be the most damaging disruption in the history of American education."[21]

Four years after Covid's start, many parents feel angry about those years. By then, not only had child tax credits expired that previously had sent monthly checks to families, but also many millions had expired that subsidized daycare centers, many of which had nonetheless failed. One woman, by profession a public defender, spent months in New Jersey arguing with officials to reopen schools. She still feels angry about those years: "I feel like Trump was a mess and Biden was a coward about doing what was right for kids. There were no grown-ups wiling to speak for what the kids needed."[22]

Four years after Covid forced schools to close, data from the Stanford Education Data Archive and the Covid-19 School Data Hub showed that "there is broad acknowledgement among many public health and education experts that extended school closures did not significantly stop the spread of Covid, while the academic harms for children have been large and long-lasting."[23]

In the obtuse language of bureaucrats, the report emphasized that with pandemics in the future, "it is to be hoped that school and public health officials will not base their decisions on fear but, in evaluating trade-offs, on epidemiological data as it emerges." In other words, don't hurt kids until you know that closing schools helps everyone.

What Have We Done to the Children?

At the end of the movie *The Bridge on the River Kwai*, Colonel Nicholson, played by Alec Guinness, has the epiphany that in building his bridge, he has helped the enemy. Fortunately, in the movie he is allowed to fall on a switch and blow up the bridge that he built.

Unfortunately, we lack a switch to undo the damage to children we inflicted. Perhaps the most unheralded damage, four years later, is the appalling rate of chronic absenteeism in schools. The *New York Times* editorial board in 2024 cited a study by the Associated Press and Stanford University documenting rates of chronic absenteeism among K–12 students, which jumped from 15 percent before the pandemic to 25 percent in the 2021–2022 school year, or an additional 6.5 million students: students who may never graduate and whose lifetime earnings will be substantially reduced. In poorer school districts such as in Oakland, California, chronic absenteeism topped 60 percent.

A follow-up study in 2024 discovered that chronic absenteeism of children in 2023 had jumped to 26 percent, compared to

15 percent before Covid.[24] The study surveyed absenteeism in forty states and the District of Columbia. In the poorest school districts, chronic absenteeism soared to nearly one-third of students.

When they are chronically absent from school, bad things happen to kids. During Covid and among adolescents aged ten to fourteen, suicide was the second-leading cause of death, and among college students aged twenty to twenty-four, suicides increased the largest amount in twenty years.[25]

Worse, with time on their hands and sometimes no supervision, homicides between teenagers jumped about 50 percent. In 2021, the combination of suicides and homicides among young people hit a twenty-year high.[26] Like excess deaths, we don't need to specify the exact causes, although we know it wasn't Covid, but we do know that lockdowns during these years were associated with a dramatic increase in depression, alienation, and hopelessness in teenagers.

Conclusions

So many kids left school for so long that they never came back. Was it worth it? Did it save lives? It doesn't appear so. Perhaps we can learn from our mistakes.

Kids in the top public- and private-school systems in America weren't harmed by extended lockdowns. Alas, most kids in America aren't lucky enough to be enrolled in great schools, so they are the ones who are now most behind and who were most harmed. And because their teachers feared getting Covid so much and went along with extended lockdowns, the kids who were harmed had few advocates.

To return to the theme about collective memory of traumatic events, who will write the history of Covid and kids' education? Historians whose children went to great schools and whose children suffered little damage? Who will be the witness for the great masses of inner-city children years left behind in math and reading, or chronically absent? Most likely, their experiences and those of their parents will not be chronicled.

NOTES

1. CDC, "COVID-19 Mortality Update—United States, 2022," May 5, 2023.

2. J. D. Sachs et al., "The Lancet Commission on Lessons for the Future from the COVID19 Pandemic," *Lancet*, vol. 400, no. 10359 (2022): 1224–80.

3. Monica Gandhi, *Endemic: A Post-Pandemic Playbook*, Mayo Clinic Press, 35.

4. Ibid., 6.

5. Ibid., 111–18.

6. Ibid.

7. Ibid.

8. Ibid., 35.

9. Johanna Sandlund et al., "Child mask mandates for COVID-19: a systematic review," *British Medical Journal*, December 3, 2023.

10. Joe Nocera and Bethany McLean, *The Big Fail: What the Pandemic Revealed about Who America Protects and Who It Leaves Behind*, Penguin, 2023, 231, my emphasis.

11. Natasha Singer, "Remote Class Exacerbated Inequalities, Report Says," *New York Times*, September 23, 2023, B1–B4.

12. Kaya Jimenz, "Covid Set Half of US Kids Behind," *USA Today*, February 3, 2023, A1.

13. Joe Nocera and Bethany McLean, *The Big Fail*, 227.

14. Paul Offit, "The Next Pandemic," *National Geographic*, February 2024, 19.

15. Natala Mehlman Petrzela, "Overzealous Measures Are Hurting Education," *Chronicle of Higher Education*, October 28, 2022, 29–32.

16. Laura Meckler, "'A Band of Tornadoes': Pandemic Hit Students Unevenly," *Washington Post*, November 24, 2022, A3.

17. Emily Oster, cited in Meckler.

18. Emily Oster, "Schools Aren't Super-Spreaders," *Atlantic*, October 9, 2020.

19. T. Cowger et al., "Lifting Universal Masking in Schools; COVID-19 Incidence Among Students and Staff," *New England Journal of Medicine*, 387:21, November 24, 2022, 1935.

20. Emily Oster, "Let's Declare a Pandemic Amnesty," *Atlantic*, October 31, 2022.

21. Editorial, *New York Times*, November 19, 2023.

22. Lisa Lerer et al., "COVID Malaise Is Killing Trust in U.S. Politics," *New York Times*, March 25, 2024, A16.

23. Sarah Mervosh et al., "Pandemic School Closures Came at a Steep Cost to Students, Data Shows," *New York Times*, March 29, 2024, A13.

24. Sarah Mervosh and Francesca Pais, "Pandemic Effect: Absence from Schools Is Soaring," *New York Times*, March 30, 2024, A1.

25. CDC, "Disparities in Suicide (by Age)," https://www.cdc.gov/suicide/facts/disparities-in-suicide.html#age.

26. Editorial, "The Main Lockdown Casualties: Children," *Wall Street Journal*, June 16, 2023.

Who Should Live When Not All Can?

Before Covid, bioethicists and medical scholars had published extensively about how to allocate scarce medical resources during pandemics. But most publications assumed a rational system in which people agreed on standards, which did not occur during Covid. As we will see, previous scholarship created some background for allocation during Covid, but it also created some problems. Covid also created unanticipated ethical issues, such as the allocation and withdrawal of ECMO (ExtraCorporeal Membrane Oxygenation) machines.

SOCIAL WORTH

The 1962 "God Committee" in Seattle, Washington, famously debated which patients should receive hemodialysis machines, which then were experimental. After screening for medical incompatibility, it allowed nonmedical values to influence selection, such as having dependent children.

This committee motivated Nicholas Rescher's 1969 paper "Allocation of Exotic Lifesaving Therapy,"[1] in which he argued that a first cut should exclude those who would not medically benefit.

Rescher then advocated additional criteria: expected years on the resource, number of dependents, and contributions to society.

When candidates came out equally, he favored a lottery. For both the God Committee and Rescher, critics called these non-medical standards "social worth" criteria.

Bioethicist James Childress's 1970 essay, "Who Shall Live When Not All Can?" argued from a Kantian perspective that medicine should reject social worth criteria.[2] Boston University law professor George Annas agreed, famously quipping that a lonely Thoreau or a prostitute would not get a machine under such standards.[3] Rescher's followers replied that they were not classifying moral worth but trying to get maximal value from scarce resources. Childress replied that human lives were being discussed here, not tools in hardware stores.

This discussion influenced states later that formulated guidelines for the allocation of ventilators or ICU beds during crises, where the criterion of medical success loomed large and where anything about social worth was suspect.

BIOETHICS AND ABLEISM

Before Covid, Alabama and Washington State had guidelines rejecting patients for scarce ventilators who had "intellectual disability or complex neurological problems."[4] At Covid's beginning, advocates for people with intellectual disabilities successfully argued before the Office of Civil Rights of Health and Human Services that these guidelines violated the Americans with Disabilities Act of 1992, so Alabama and Washington State abolished their guidelines. Importantly, this Office also stated that hospitals should not exclude patients because of advanced age.

In 2015, New York State's Task Force on Life and the Law developed Sequential Organ Failure Assessment (SOFA) scores to prioritize ventilator allocation.[5] Bioethicist Joseph Fins and the late disability advocate Adrienne Asch worried that crypto-discrimination against people with disabilities, such as heart conditions associated with Down syndrome, might mask unjust screening, but have no bearing on survival.

SOFA evaluates how critical organs (liver, kidney, heart, lungs) perform and scores the functions of each organ. Patients with high SOFA scores were most likely to die. SOFA scores were developed for patients with sepsis, and for them SOFA scores are accurate: "If 100 severely ill septic patients requiring intensive care unit treatment have a SOFA score greater than 11, over 90% of them will die."[6] At the start of Covid, SOFA scores were important.

In the first year of Covid, physician Ezekiel Emanuel of the University of Pennsylvania emerged on cable television and in op-ed essays as a leading bioethicist willing to speak about Covid. When medical personnel were forced to choose who would get a ventilator or who would get admitted to an ICU, Emanuel argued for maximizing life-years.[7] So give a scarce, lifesaving machine to a forty-year-old, not some eighty-year-old. Emanuel's recommendation contradicted directions of the Office of Civil Rights not to exclude the elderly.

In sum, at Covid's start, two criteria became important in allocating scarce medical resources: (1) expected medical prognosis, especially prognosis based on SOFA scores, and (2) exclusion both of social worth evaluations and rationing based on age or disabilities.

STRUCTURAL PROBLEMS

One unanticipated ethical issue about allocation concerned significant inequalities among American hospitals. Wealthier hospitals had better staffing, resources, and funding than poorer hospitals. In New York City, NYU's Langone Medical Center had far better resources than Brooklyn's King's County or Maimonides Hospitals. In Alabama, UAB Medical Center had far more resources, including pulmonary physicians and specialists in infectious diseases, than community hospitals. When you got sick with Covid, where you went determined a lot about how you fared.

Another structural problem was that virtually every small hospital in America had a catheterization lab and an orthopedic surgery program for knee and hip replacements, but they didn't have ICUs. If you measure the number of rooms in a hospital devoted to orthopedic and cardiovascular procedures versus ICU beds for critically ill people, American hospitals had changed from places that took care of sick people to places that performed lucrative procedures.

UAB hospitals during Covid's peak had four hundred Covid patients and about twelve ICU units. Overall, it had 1,100 total beds, some of which were converted to ICU beds. During that surge, elderly patients often died quickly, both in ICUs and in regular rooms. But some patients lasted a long time, and for them, decisions needed to be made about keeping them for months on ECMO.

ECMO

Most people understand ventilators, which have been used for over sixty years, and which force air through a tube placed in the trachea into the lungs, expanding them. When the lungs deflate, the ventilator sucks carbon dioxide out of lungs before the next cycle begins. Ventilators can quickly deliver extra oxygen to patients and don't need as much staffing as ECMO, but they usually necessitate heavy sedation.

When Covid severely damaged a patient's lungs, ventilators could not produce good levels of oxygenated blood, and so ECMO became a possibility. ECMO uses a membrane oxygenator (aka "artificial lung") to infuse blood with oxygen and remove carbon dioxide. Surgeons sometimes put patients on ECMO, attaching tubes to major veins or arteries so blood can flow safely outside the body. (If ECMO machines are unfamiliar to you, watching a YouTube video may be helpful.)[8]

Surgeons first developed ECMO for children. Prior to Covid, ECMO was sometimes a last resort for adults waiting for heart transplants.

ECMO machines did not need to be used in ICU rooms, creating a logistical advantage in some hospitals. Patients could be awake on ECMO, which was good if they couldn't tolerate the tracheal tube needed for a ventilator. When they regained some lung function, patients could walk while still connected to an ECMO machine.

One downside, however, is that if ECMO machines malfunction, patients cannot breathe on their own, and they die instantly. And Covid patients who spent months on ECMO machines emerged with very weak overall muscle strength.

Importantly, because ECMO is a last resort for critically ill patients, and because it's at best a halfway measure, only half of the patients put on it survive. Also, because it requires monitoring twenty-four hours a day, every day, and because it can cause infections and blood clots, ECMO is mainly used in academic medical centers with specialists on staff. Most small community hospitals lack ECMO machines or the trained staff to use them.

Seattle ECLS Consortium

ECMO was a new, expensive, complex option for pulmonary doctors, one whose allocation created new ethical issues during Covid. The Seattle Ethics in ECLS Consortium identified several ethical issues involving ECMO with "Betty's case."[9] Betty was "an obese, unvaccinated, previously healthy 22-year-old Covid patient" with severe respiratory distress syndrome and complex pneumonia, for whom ventilators had failed to supply enough oxygen, so she went on ECMO. Due to staff shortages, administrators transferred her to a pediatric ICU for ECMO for four weeks, followed by three weeks intubated on a ventilator. The Consortium worried that during Betty's seven weeks there, critically ill children who were then diverted to other places did not get optimal care.

The Seattle ECLS group identified other ethical issues about who received ECMO: ambiguity about who makes decisions, urgency of decisions needing to be made in life-or-death moments, uncertain prognoses fraught with possible serious complications, diverse populations of varying health status, large medical teams with differing opinions, and disputes about "national and international guidelines based on expert opinion {see the Delphi group below} rather than on clinical data."

THE SELECTION OF ECMO PATIENTS AND THEIR DURATION ON ECMO

Prior to Covid, little consensus existed about the selection of patients for ECMO, or when better candidates arrived, about how long patients with a poor prognosis should be continued on ECMO.

During the most intense surges of Covid, hospitals with limited ECMO machines encountered dozens of patients needing the only one remaining machine, and they then had to decide whom to save. To discover best practices in such a situation, a Delphi study in 2020 convened twenty-two international experts, each with at least five years' experience with ECMO patients.[10]

This Delphi group did not think SOFA scores were relevant, but they did think age and multiple medical problems were exclusionary criteria:

> *Currently, there is no evidence-based scoring system to guide ECMO prioritization during resource limitations. However, factors predicting poor outcomes may be utilized to prioritize patients for ECMO.*
>
> *Rationale: Due to a lack of resources, ethical dilemmas regarding patient prioritization for ECMO pose unique challenges. Patients may be prioritized for ECMO treatment*

based on factors that predict poor outcomes. Increasing age, multiple comorbidities, and cumulative organ failures are the most common predictors of mortality and may determine which patients receive priority for ECMO.

The first sentence implicitly disputes using SOFA scores to predict prognosis the of Covid patients on ECMO. This is important because Chelen et al. surveyed allocation documents in twenty academic medical centers and found that use of SOFA scores "was the most common criterion of triage in 19 (95%) of 20 policies."[11]

The Delphi group spotted this problem because Covid patients usually had severe lung impairment, but their other organs might be normal, so their SOFA score might be only 4 to 5 where scores of 10 to 11 were exclusionary. The National Academies of Sciences, Engineering, and Medicine agreed, saying SOFA scores for Covid patients were "poor predictors of individual patients' survival, particularly those with primary respiratory failure."[12]

Like many allocation issues during Covid, and given this problem with SOFA scores and the chaos in some hospitals during Covid surges, it is unclear what actually happened.

Another consensus by the Delphi group emphasized a specific age range during a surge of patients for selection:

During a surge in patient volume, the cutoff age could vary worldwide depending on ECMO capacity and resource availability. As a result, we advise setting the cutoff age in a national or regional policy, if needed, due to limited resources.

Rationale: Age is strongly associated with patient outcomes and should be considered during patient selection. All cohorts of ECMO in Covid-19 that studied predictors of mortality retained age in their regression analysis model, and the median age or age grouping was approximately 45–55 years.

[my emphasis] It is crucial to distinguish between numerical age and biological age.

But implying that patients over the age of fifty-five could be excluded raised alarms because the Office of Civil Rights had forbidden this. But many intensivists wondered: What did some faceless bureaucrat in Washington know about his dilemmas with ECMO patients?

It appears that many institutions altered their documents to comply. Nevertheless, it is unclear what happened, especially because advanced age with multiple comorbidities usually predicted poor outcomes for Covid patients in ICU beds, on ventilators, or on ECMO.

ETHICS ISSUES ABOUT ECMO NEEDING FURTHER STUDY

Covid patients who received ECMO came from all kinds of backgrounds with many different problems. While on ECMO, some were susceptible to clots, heart failure, or immune system failure.[13] Many had acute respiratory distress syndrome (ARDS). Even for the half who survived, their long-term prognosis was (and still is) unclear.

Several policies surveyed by Chelen's group found that some hospital policies used a version of social worth criteria: some prioritized medical workers; others prioritized essential workers (police, firefighters, and emergency responders). Again, although Americans generally agreed that essential workers should be vaccinated first, did they also agree about saving them first? Let's hope so. Chelen's group also just surveyed *policies*, not whether such policies were followed or were good.

Inappropriate use of ECMO, such as a "never-give-up-on-anybody" attitude, led to some bad outcomes. If ECMO was denied to someone who might have lived with it because the wrong person got the machine, that is bad. Second, one study found that ECMO was unsuccessful in 54 percent of Covid adults with ARDS, but only 30 percent of adults who had a cardiac arrest.[14] For the latter patient on ECMO, did giving him ECMO merely extend his suffering?

As said, half of patients on ECMO failed to survive. As this fact became known, pulmonary doctors wondered if utilizing ECMO was a good strategy at all, because it was linked to iatrogenic infections, and for some patients, it merely prolonged the inevitable. For some intensivists, whether to put patients on ECMO stressed them more than allocating ICU beds or ventilators.

OTHER ETHICAL ISSUES ABOUT ECMO

It is one thing to turn ICU beds on the cardiac or surgery floors into units for Covid patients, or put more people on ECMO, but is that a good thing? What happens when other surgical patients need treatment? Some such types of surgery can be postponed or delayed, but not all of them. What about the critically ill children who could not get good care because Betty was being treated in their facility? Does it make sense for several staff to care for an ECMO patient while dozens of others cannot get scheduled operations?

For interventional cardiologists, being assigned to care for ECMO patients could be frustrating when their normal cardiac patients cannot get treated. Some patients in their eighties with a predicted survival of nine months to two years without surgery nevertheless delayed surgery for fear of getting Covid or because rooms or surgeons were unavailable.

WITHDRAWING VERSUS FOREGOING

What about the difference between not putting patients on ECMO versus withdrawing them from it? This illustrates the acting-omitting distinction in bioethics, also called withdrawing versus foregoing. Of course, discontinuing devices from patients when it will quickly lead to death feels different from omitting lifesaving treatment. An extensive literature in bioethics discusses this topic, dating back to the seminal article by James Rachels.[15] For ECMO, several policies emphasized reassessment and "retriage timing" of ECMO patients, which implied "decannulation" for failing patients.

Rationing ECMO

The rationing of ECMO machines certainly occurred during Covid. Even something as simple as obtaining more ECMO catheters became a flashpoint when they were unavailable, or when the hospital was unwilling to pay inflated prices for them. Hospitals using ECMO ran out of beds and indirectly rationed by denying transfers from less-well-equipped hospitals.

In a revealing study about the pandemic's most intense months, Whitney Gannon and colleagues at Vanderbilt University discovered that because of a lack of ECMO machines and staffing there, nearly 90 percent of adult Covid-19 patients who were eligible for ECMO did not receive it and died in the hospital. "Eligible" meant they were under sixty years old, not morbidly obese, and had failed a ventilator trial, but they were otherwise healthy.[16]

The median age of those eligible was forty. The Vanderbilt hospital could handle thirty-five patients on ECMO, but they had 240 referred for it. "Even when saving ECMO for the youngest, healthiest and sickest patients, we could only provide it to a fraction of patients who qualified for it," said Gannon. "I hope these data encourage hospitals and federal authorities to invest in the capacity to provide ECMO to more patients."[17] A physician involved in the study said, "This data suggests that, on average, providing ECMO to two patients will save a life and give a young person the potential to live for decades."[18]

Despite Gannon's plea, before American repeats its experience with scarce hemodialysis machines—which caused Congress to pass the End Stage Renal Disease Act funding dialysis for every American—further study needs to be done about who benefits, and who does not, from ECMO.

Gannon's plea also raises a larger question of values about investing in expensive machines for cardiac failure, such as artificial hearts, left-ventricle assist (LVAD) machines, and ECMO. Is such investment justified when tens of millions of Americans, because of lack of medical insurance, lack access to primary, preventive care?

FINAL NOTE

In researching this book, I found it difficult to get physicians to talk on the record about allocation decisions made during Covid. Many reasons exist for this. As one told me, "I just want to forget those terrible years." Another said something similar: "The chaos of Covid's first year was unbelievable: the story needs to be told, but not by me."

In America, doctors fear being sued for malpractice, so that makes them reluctant to talk about hard cases. Because the Office of Civil Rights decision forbade the exclusion of eighty-five-year-olds with dementia, it is now difficult for anyone to talk about doing so during Covid.

The isolation protocols surrounding Covid patients in hospitals also meant that families could not visit sick relatives, nor could physicians talk to families in person. Instead, many communicated by phone or through glass windows. This did not facilitate trust. Some suspicious families posted comments about physicians on social media, often out of context or in disparaging ways, further eroding trust.

Also, alas, facts about Covid became politicized, also eroding trust between doctors and the families of patients. Some families would not accept that Covid was real or that their father had it, much less that their father had died of it. Others, following Donald Trump's suggestion, demanded prescriptions for ivermectin.

I empathize with physicians who feared angry families suspecting discrimination and seeing the physicians treating their relatives not as heroes but as adversaries. As one told me, "If I'm risking my life for my Covid patients, I need them to be grateful."

So many unexpected ethical issues arose that trying to anticipate them is like the old folly of medieval casuistry. For example, over eight weeks in the spring of 2020 in New York City, bioethicist Joseph Fins and his ethics consultants were on call 24/7 supporting nurses, residents, and unit chiefs, "providing 2500 ethics consultations and addressing a range of horrific questions they'd never previously considered," such as whether to withhold CPR from a dying Covid patient without a signed DNR order, which was required by New York law, or whether to allow infectious Covid patients to leave for places where they lived close to others.[19]

Because America lacked clear, transparent criteria about how to allocate medical resources, doctors and administrators were often on their own. Although they might have conferred with other institutions or used hospital ethics committees to create guidelines, they ultimately had to make tough decisions by themselves and felt, as one told me, that "no one had my back."

As a result, it may take years to find out exactly how ventilators, ECMO machines, and other scarce medical resources were distributed during Covid. That is sad, because we need to know what happened to establish better policies in the future. In 1996, at the end of apartheid in South Africa, Nelson Mandela convened the Truth and Reconciliation Commission to discuss what happened and why. Perhaps we need a similar commission to discuss what happened during Covid. Otherwise, we may be in danger of returning to the 1950s, when medicine had an internal, private ethics unshared with the public.[20]

The SARS1 pandemic in 2009 created a decade of patients needing ECMO; we can anticipate that SARS2 will do the same.

This is especially true for the millions of Americans with Long Covid, so the ethical issues raised by ECMO continue.

The use of age in triaging patients remains a key ethical issue. A forty-eight-year-old had a much better chance of success on ECMO, especially on a limited trial, than an eighty-five-year-old. This issue needs much further discussion because, yes, let's take the eighty-five-year-old off ECMO and give it to a fifty-five-year-old, but what if that person fares poorly and a thirty-five-year-old enters who also needs ECMO? How far do you go with younger patients, and how many times? Do the nonmedical characteristics of needy patients matter at all? What if the patient was sixty-seven-year-old pulmonary physician who became infected after a year of treating Covid patients?

If there is such a thing as an "under the table" bioethical issue, the allocation of ECMO machines during Covid was one. This is not a problem of different collective memories, but rather, a problem yet to be recognized. Deciding how people live and die should not be an internal decision of doctors, but one with publicly-agreed-upon standards. We can achieve this, but first the problem needs to be bought out in the open.

NOTES

1. Nicholas Rescher, "The Allocation of Exotic Lifesaving Therapy," *Ethics* 79, April 1969.

2. James Childress, "Who Shall Live When Not All Can Live?" *Soundings* 53, 1970.

3. George Annas, "The Prostitute, the Playboy, and the Poet: Rationing Schemes for Organ Transplantation," *American Journal of Public Health* 75, no. 3 (1985), 187–89.

4. Johnny Kampis, "Alabama's Pandemic Emergency Plan Discriminates Against People with Disabilities," *Tuscaloosa News*, March 31, 2020.

5. Joseph Fins, "Disabusing the Disability Critique of the New York State Task Force Report on Ventilator Allocation," April 1, 2020, *Hastings Bioethics Forum.*

6. "SOFA Score: What It Is and How to Use It in Triage," TRACIE: Healthcare Emergency Preparedness Gateway. Some scholars thought SOFA mimicked existing practice during COVID, but they thought

it could be tweaked: D. Anderson et al., "Rationing Scarce Healthcare Capacity: A Study of the Ventilator Allocation Guidelines during the COVID-19 Pandemic," *Productions and Operation Management*, Special Issue, December 3, 2022.

7. Ezekiel J. Emanuel et al., "Fair Allocation of Scarce Medical Resources in the Time of COVID," *New England Journal of Medicine*, May 21, 2020, 382: 2049–55.

8. For example, https://www.youtube.com/watch?v=jl_y4Sj9ht0.

9. Joanna Clark et al., "Ethical Considerations in Ever-Expanding Utilization of ECLS: A Research Agenda," *Frontiers of Pediatrics*, May 19, 2022: 10:896232.

10. Ahmed Rabie et al., "Expert consensus statement on venovenous extracorporeal membrane oxygenation ECMO for COVID-19 severe ARDS: an international Delphi study," *Annals of Intensive Care*, 20243: 13:36, published May 2, 2023, doi: 10.1186/s13613-023-01126-9.

11. Julia Chelen et al., "Use of Ventilator Allocation and Patient Triage Policies in Anticipation of the COVID-19 Surge," *Health Security*, vol. 19, no. 5, 2021.

12. National Academies of Sciences, Engineering, Washington, DC: The National Academies Press; 2020, accessed May 4, 2021, https://doi.org/10.17226/25765.

13. Heinsar et al., "ECMO during the COVID-19 pandemic: When is it justified?" *Critical Care*, vol. 24, 2020.

14. Joanna Clark et al., "Ethical Considerations in Ever-Expanding Utilization of ECLS: A Research Agenda," *Frontiers of Pediatrics*, May 19, 2022: 10:896232.

15. James Rachels, "Active and Passive Euthanasia," *New England Journal of Medicine*, January 9, 1975, vol. 292, no. 2: 78, doi: 10.1056/NEJM197501092920206.

16. Mary Van Beusekom, "Study: 90% of young ECMO-eligible COVID patients at a US hospital died amid rationing," *American Journal of Respiratory and Critical Care Medicine*, CIDRAP News, February 28, 2022.

17. Whitney Gannon, quoted in Vanderbilt University Medical Center, news release: "Study shows young, healthy adults died from COVID-19 due to ECMO shortage," February 25, 2022; Whitney Gannon, "Association between Availability of Extracorporeal Membrane Oxygenation and Mortality in Patients with COVID-19 Eligible for Extracorporeal Membrane Oxygenation: A Natural Experiment," *American Journal of Respiratory and Critical Care Medicine*, vol. 205, no. 11.

18. Jonathan Casey, MD, quoted in above news release.

19. Jordan Kisner, "The Committee on Life and Death," *Atlantic*, January–February 2021, 40.

20. Carl Elliott recently wrote about this problem: "In Medicine, the Morally Unthinkable Too Easily Comes to Seem Normal," *New York Times*, May 7, 2024.

CHAPTER 5

Some Philosophical Questions
Raised by Pandemics

Pandemics raise many philosophical questions, certainly more than most people conceptualize as philosophical. To set the stage for the chapters to come, what follows is a brief discussion of such questions.

WHO IS AN "ESSENTIAL WORKER"?

Consider the question, Who is an essential worker? During Covid, various organizations suggested that essential workers should be the first to get vaccinated. Of course, *should* is also a value word.

Most scholars and everyday people agreed that, as essential workers, doctors and nurses on the front lines should get vaccinated first. During a pandemic, they constituted the most essential of all essential workers. If they all became sick at the same time, the medical system would collapse.

However, this idea became controversial when physicians and nurses *not* on the front lines wanted to be vaccinated first. Especially annoying were those who worked from home, such as radiologists viewing MRI scans from the safety of offices in their basements, yet who still wanted to be vaccinated ahead of cashiers in grocery stores. Some even pretended they were frontline workers, but they were exposed by real frontline medical workers who used their cell phones to photograph them in line and shamed them on social media.

Once we vaccinate all frontline doctors and nurses, the question is, Who comes next? Bus drivers on city routes? Police officers? Firefighters? Teachers of K–12 children? Airline pilots and flight attendants? TSA screeners at airports? Workers on assembly lines in large plants making cars or cutting up cows, all of whom work closely together and interact frequently? No clear answer can easily be found, especially when it implies to other groups that they are "nonessential."

WHAT IS "CONTAGIOUS"?

Consider contagion, which we usually think of only in terms of germs, yet those who study the prevention of injuries and deaths think of contagion more broadly. For example, in 2015, 25 percent of gun murders occurred in neighborhoods that compose less than 2 percent of America's population.[1] Can murder in such neighborhoods be considered "contagious"?

Some epidemiologists discuss how well-publicized stories about a suicide can create a spike in suicides afterward.[2] Are copycat killers examples of psychopathological contagion? Do sociopathic people exist who yearn for public attention and resent the attention of a publicized serial killer, so they then kill the same way? In 1888, the real Jack the Ripper in London received great attention, and such attention seems to have spawned similar killings, creating the phrase "copycat killer." In 1982 in America, someone killed seven people in Chicago with Extra Strength Tylenol tablets laced with cyanide, a crime that spurred similar poisonings in other cities. The number of copycat killers in America is painful to continue listing, but the curious can follow this endnote.[3]

Political philosophers might go even further and claim that despotic behavior can be contagious, citing how the rise of Vladimir Putin in Russia and China's Xi Jinping created copycats such as Erdogan in Turkey, Nicolás Maduro in Venezuela, Kim Jong Un in North Korean, Narendra Modi in India, and Donald Trump in the United States.

A more troubling question concerns whether bad leadership can be contagious. The outlandish political style of Donald Trump seemed contagious in America, creating wannabes such as former New York City mayor Rudy Giuliani, senator Josh Hawley, congressman Matt Gaetz, and congresswoman Marjorie Taylor Greene, all of whom seem to have abandoned all ethical principles. And then there was Jair Bolsonaro in Brazil, who seemed to pattern his behavior after Trump, adopting the strongman posture during Covid and acting as if it were unmanly to fear an invisible virus.

Even more broadly, can vice be outrageous? In an unjust society, is selfish, greedy behavior contagious? Plato implied that it can be.

One of the hardest lessons we've learned in the last century concerns how we often fail to understand the changes caused by new technology, such as the internal combustion engine's effect on the climate. Similarly, we underestimated the power of social media—including Facebook, Instagram, and TikTok—to influence behavior. In pandemics, we have paid special attention to amplification systems that accelerated the spread of germs, say in days from a few people to a few thousand. Is social media now an amplification system for bad behavior, making ethnic tribalism, racism, and antisemitism contagious?

In general, it seems too narrow-minded to assume that only germs can be contagious. Contagion more broadly is a much more interesting philosophical concept.[4]

Who Is Most Vulnerable?

Consider another philosophical problem, this time concerning the protection of society's most vulnerable people. Harvard philosopher John Rawls famously argued that a just society protects its most vulnerable members. During Covid, the most vulnerable people to sickness and death from the virus were those living closely together in "congregate living facilities," such as homeless shelters, prisons, and mental health institutions. Should they have been vaccinated first? Should they have been among the most protected?

Alas, vaccinating people without homes before voting citizens might not be practical in real democracies. Pandemics breed fear, and fear makes people tribal and selfish, as we will see with international efforts to vaccinate the poor (see chapter 13).

The Covid pandemic exposed structural inequalities in the United States that terribly hurt minorities and vulnerable groups. People of color often worked face-to-face with customers, such as bus drivers, nursing home aides, grocery store cashiers, long-haul truckers, construction workers, and cleaning staff. Unsurprisingly, many such workers were paid hourly, often deliberately less than forty hours a week so employers weren't required to give them medical insurance. To keep their families fed, they had to work and interact with many other people, and as such, they suffered a high percentage of Covid infections.

And Covid deaths. In Illinois, Black Americans made up 14 percent of that state's population, but half of its Covid deaths.[5] Noam Chomsky emphasized these themes and points out that although Blacks are 32 percent of Louisiana's citizens, they accounted for 70 percent of its Covid deaths. Overall, Chomsky concluded, "These figures reflect the fact that lower-income African Americans do not have the same ability to protect themselves through social distancing and staying home from their jobs."[6]

And given that so many these essential workers of color were female, is it any surprise that most Long Haulers are also women? As we shall see in chapter 17, their low wages and lack of medical insurance virtually guarantees that they can't qualify for disability benefits because they probably never saw a doctor for Covid, can't afford a clinic for Long Covid, and can't document their original Covid infection.

Inhabitants of nursing homes in America were likely the most vulnerable to die from Covid infection. According to Paul Offit, MD, a vaccine expert, "older adults suffered a death rate about a thousand-fold greater than children; at times, as many as 40 percent of Covid deaths in the U.S. occurred in nursing homes."[7]

A report by health policy researchers at Harvard Medical School and the University of Rochester graded the American system of nursing homes at a D.[8] When many Americans infected with Covid immediately took monoclonal antibodies, Paxlovid, or other antiviral medicines, only 20 percent of infected patients in nursing homes got Paxlovid, which can be taken as pills over five days. Almost half of America's fifteen thousand nursing homes reported never giving their infected clients Paxlovid. Although Medicare or Medicaid or the CARES Act would have paid for this medication, the lack of staff, coupled with the need for social and physical distancing, prevented such treatments.

Prisoners were also leading candidates for being the most vulnerable to death from Covid, and America incarcerates more people per capita than any other country in the world.[9] Deaths in prisons during 2020 saw a 50 percent increase.[10] These figures mostly continued through 2021. In six states, death rates doubled from 2020 to 2021. Thus, focusing on prisons should be a logical priority in protecting those most vulnerable to death from Covid.

But vaccinating prisoners before ordinary citizens proved politically risky. Critics claimed that because prisoners had committed crimes, and despite where and how they were housed, they did not deserve to be vaccinated before most other citizens. In Colorado, Governor Jared Polis ignored recommendations of his own commission to vaccinate prisoners first.

The most vulnerable of all were poor women with children in developing countries. Risks of infectious diseases, like Covid, AIDS, or severe diarrhea, force impossible decisions on families about working versus staying home. According to UNICEF, in the two years after 2019, one hundred million more children fell into poverty, a 10 percent increase.[11]

CONCLUSIONS

Many key terms or phrases in thinking about pandemics and their ethical issues are ambiguous. Previously, we discussed different kinds of immunity from vaccines and different meanings of the term *herd immunity*. Add to that list differing meanings of *essential workers*, *contagious behavior*, and the *most vulnerable people to infectious diseases*.

NOTES

1. Adam Kucharski, *The Rules of Contagion*, Basic Books, 2020, 123.

2. Ibid., 122.

3. "10 Notable Copycat Killers," *How Stuff Works*, https://people. howstuffworks.com/5-copycat-killers.htm.

4. This discussion is heavily indebted to Kuchaski's excellent book *The Rules of Contagion*.

5. C. J. Polychroniou, "Interviews with Noam Chomsky," *Precipice*, Haymarket Books, 2021, 280.

6. Ibid.

7. Paul Offit, "The Next Pandemic," *National Geographic*, February 2024, 19.

8. Paula Span, "How Nursing Homes Failed on COVID Protection," *New York Times*, August 22, 2023.

9. Emily Widra and Tiana Herring, "States of Incarceration: The Global Context 2021," Prison Policy Initiative, September 2021, https:// www.prisonpolicy.org/global/2021.html.

10. J. Valentino-DeVries and Allie Pitchon, "As COVID Gripped US, Death Swept Through Prisons," *New York Times*, February 19, 2023.

11. DefeatDD, "Carrying Children through COVID-19 and Beyond," https://www.defeatdd.org/campaign/carrying-children-through-COVID -19-and-beyond?gad_source=5&gclid=EAIaIQobChMIqN_D-cvsgwMV X1tHAR1xQAIMEAAYBSAAEgK85PD_BwE.

Chapter 6

Investigating Covid's Origins

Because some readers may think the origins of Covid are well-established and that alternative explanations are all political propaganda, they may be tempted to skip this chapter. I hope they do not. If nothing else, it will dispel the notion that Covid's origins are settled. This chapter also illustrates this book's themes about suppression of unpopular views and the consequent distrust of public officials. The problems it identifies also bode ill for international cooperation in containing new viruses.

The prevailing official theory is that SARS2 came as a crossover virus from a wet market in Wuhan, but this theory has several problems. First, SARS2 looks like a bat virus, and live bats weren't for sale in that market. Second, a famous Chinese virologist, Shi Zhengli, worked on bat viruses in the nearby Wuhan Institute of Virology. Third, destroying the wet market to remove any remnants of SARS2 was seen by some as wiping a crime scene. Fourth, Chinese authorities continue to block any investigation by international scientists of the origins of SARS2.

Christopher Wray, the former director of the FBI, told the world in 2022 that, "The FBI has for quite some time now assessed that the origins of the pandemic are most likely a potential lab incident in Wuhan."[1] This is the same FBI director whose conclusions are taken seriously by Congress, by reporters, and by the American public when he warns of dangers of interference in elections by China and Russia, about members of ISIS slipping across America's southern border, and about cybercrimes.

Wray's statement fueled speculation as to whether the FBI learned something about Covid's origins from intercepted messages from spying on China or from some mole inside China. The US Department of Energy came to the same conclusion, agreeing with Wray about a lab leak.

While the CIA, whose main responsibility is to investigate issues such as this, officially rejects the lab-leak theory, its denial has been controversial. According to *Science* magazine, an anonymous whistleblower inside the CIA told the congressional panel investigating a lab leak that the CIA had "bribed" six CIA analysts to reject the lab-leak theory. A press release said, "The House's Permanent Select Committee on Intelligence have heard testimony from a whistleblower 'who presents as a highly credible senior-level CIA officer.' . . . The whistleblower testified that only the most senior analyst of a seven-member CIA team investigating the origin of Covid-19 supported the zoonotic transmission theory. The whistleblower alleged the other six team members supporting the lab origin then received 'a significant monetary incentive to change their position.'"[2]

One physician who believes in the lab-leak theory is Francis Sweeny, host of the popular podcast *Straight Talk MD*.[3] Sweeny, along with virologist Jonathan Lathan, whom Sweeny interviews, both believe that getting to the truth about the origins of SARS2 is "the most important story in the world now," especially if we care about preventing future pandemics.

One thing seems true both then and now: There is no consensus among scientists about the origins of SARS2. It is a "false narrative" to claim that there is such a consensus that SARS2 was a "natural zoonosis transmission" from an animal market in Wuhan. A significant number of respected scientists and journalists believe that SARS2 originated from gain-of-function research in the Wuhan lab and that a modified virus from that lab inadvertently got out.

I have witnessed nothing quite like this in fifty years of covering science writers. On one side, famous science writers such as British journalist Nicholas Wade and *New York Times* science writer Donald McNeil Jr. believe something happened in a lab in Wuhan that helped create the highly infectious coronavirus SARS-COV-2. They also hint that in an online meeting of famous evolutionary virologists, Anthony Fauci and Francis Collins tried to quash any lab-leak theories. McNeil alleges that famous virologists such as Edward Holmes, Kristian Anderson, and Andrew Rambaut deliberately misled him away from lab-manipulation theories, a claim they reject.[4]

On the other side, certain famous virologists admit that initially they suspected manipulation of the lab in Wuhan, but then decided, based on finding a similar virus that infected pangolins, that it could have occurred naturally. Science writer David Quammen offered this idea in an early defense in 2022 of the above virologists, but he concluded that the coronavirus evolved outside a lab.[5]

Part of the above controversy involves rival definitions of a non-wildlife spillover of the virus' origins. The worst, which everyone rejects, is the deliberate creation of an infectious virus to be used as a biological or economic weapon. But what about possibilities in between that dark one and a spillover from animals sold in the market?

An interesting explanation has evolved about the lab-leak theory, one that avoids imputing dark motives to the Chinese. Nicholas Wade concluded in 2024 that, "The latest information, released last month, makes a formidable case that the virus is the product of laboratory synthesis, not of nature. This startling fact will probably take some time to sink into the national consciousness, given the mainstream media's sustained inability to report the issue objectively."[6]

Wade emphasizes the benign explanation that Chinese scientists at the now-infamous Wuhan Institute of Virology—where the "bat lady" scientist Shi Zhengli worked—were trying to prevent SARS-type viruses from crossing to humans from bats, and as such, were trying to develop a special kind of vaccine in bats for this purpose.

Wade emphasizes how in 2018, a team of American scientists, affiliated with a company called EcoHealth Alliance, applied for grants with the Chinese "Bat Lady," Shi Zhengli, to the Pentagon's DARPA [Defense Advanced Research Projects] for a fourteen-million-dollar grant to manipulate bat viruses related to SARS-COV-1. Their application, called Project DEFUSE, claimed they would enhance the infectivity of the original virus by inserting changes into a point in the genetic makeup called a furin cleavage site, and especially by using a biological restriction enzyme called BsmBI. (Eco-Health came under federal investigation in late 2023 for possibly double-billing—China and America—for the same research.)[7]

The basic point is that SARS2, which started the Covid pandemic, shows strong evidence of laboratory enhancement in ways lacking in a thousand other members of the same family of viruses. It shows changes at a furin cleavage site that used BsmBI.

Of course, Chinese virologists couldn't capture and vaccinate individual bats in caves where thousands lived, so they came up with the idea of vaccinating a few dozen founder bats with a self-spreading virus created from a bat coronavirus. So argues science journalist Jim Haslam, who believes that this "vaccine coronavirus" accidentally escaped in a worker from the lab and infected citizens of Wuhan, and then, of course, the world, as SARS2.[8]

This is not to claim that anything funded by Anthony Fauci or American scientists was involved. Nor does it claim that anything intentional happened. The Wuhan lab worked with many viruses and many bats, and the lesson here might simply be that one slip of a changed virus can affect the world.

Without going into the biochemical details, the advantage of this last explanation is that examination of SARS2 by experts reveals an amazing coincidence as to where the virus seems to have been manipulated to allow the insertion of new material. Second, if SARS2 was the result of a "natural transmission" from animals in a Wuhan animal market, after four years, one would expect similar transmissions from other wet markets in Asia, but none seems to have occurred. Finally, it has never been proven that live bats or pangolins were ever even sold in the Wuhan market.

Furthermore, as physician Ravi Iyer emphasized in his book about the Covid pandemic, most viruses that jump from bats to humans (through antigenic drift) undergo a period of adaptation in the human hosts: "It is like a dating game between a boy and a girl pairing up for the first time. The initial interactions are tentative as the virus evolves towards its best fit to its host. So, in such cases, the initial spread is hesitant and sporadic. . . . [By contrast] the SARS2 virus was behaving as if it was already well adapted to its human host."[9]

British science journalist Debora MacKenzie quotes Andrew Rambaut of the University of Edinburgh, whose specialty is viral emergence, and who discovered that the first few sequences of infected patients posted by doctors in Wuhan—before China closed the door on such postings—were "genetically identical."[10] MacKenzie argues that if the virus had jumped from animals, or had been circulating for a while in people, it would have acquired genetic variations in these early infections. Rambaut concluded in 2020, before he seems to have been pressured to conclude the other way, "I would say it was definitely a single jump, and it was probably not before early November."[11]

Nicholas Wade came to the same conclusion: "And whereas most viruses require repeated tries to switch from an animal host to people, SARS-COV-2 infected humans out of the box, as if it had been manipulated in the humanized mice called for in the DEFUSE protocol."[12]

How to explain this? One explanation is that SARS2 had been infecting humans in Wuhan for some time, but other than six miners exposed for a long time in a bat cave during September 2019, other citizens of Wuhan were not sickened, and given the virulent transmissibility of SARS2 (with a Ro coefficient of 2.4 to 4), that should have occurred. The other, more likely, explanation is that SARS2 had been created in a lab as a "human capable bat virus" that could spread fast.

Finally, a darker side exists about the lab-leak explanation. Yes, American agencies and companies had some ties to the Wuhan Institute of Virology, and they have not been forthcoming about Freedom of Information requests from journalists to release correspondence about their cooperation. If China was completely to blame for an accidental release of SARS2, why wouldn't American agencies be more transparent about their past collaborations with the Wuhan Institute of Virology? Is it possible that this is another "Spanish flu" diversion, where some research that helped create SARS2 was funded by American interests? If so, this would explain the reluctance of both China and America to vigorously pursue the origins of SARS2.

As with the effort to shut down talk of Focused Protection and to suppress rare but bad effects of Covid vaccinations, top officials claimed a false consensus about the "natural transmission" explanation from wet markets and tried to shut down the lab-leak theory. Indeed, on February 19, 2020, Peter Daszak, the president of EcoHealth Alliance, received a letter published online in the British Journal *Lancet*, signed by twenty-seven scientists, which concluded, "We stand together to strongly condemn conspiracy theories suggesting that Covid-19 does not have a natural origin."[13]

Note that this claim is made very early in 2020. Note who organized it. Note its ambiguity (perhaps a spillover from a changed bat virus to a Chinese person is a "natural origin"?). In any case, it's hard to believe that a consensus among scientists could emerge so quickly about the origins of this virus, especially given that China did not cooperate at all. Four years later, Daszak was required to testify before Congress about misrepresentations in his applications for funding of viral research with the Wuhan Institute.[14]

The result has been to make a significant number of journalists, physicians, and educated professionals distrust not only public health officials, but also virologists and other scientists. Certainly, any effort to cancel debate on this topic, which certainly occurred and is still occurring, as in "this is too complex for the public to understand," reeks of paternalism and elitism.

We saw how scientists and physicians in the public eye, as well as editors in the news media, closed ranks to suppress discussion of Focused Protection and how they earlier tried to close ranks about the value of masks, vaccinations, a spread-only-by-droplets virus, whether vaccines protected 100 percent against infection, and so on, even when the evidence forced them later to contradict themselves. So, this same group seems to have closed ranks to cancel theories about laboratory manipulation, making people think that too much of science was politicized, which— given the huge sums of money involved in big grants and the national pride—maybe it was.

CONCLUSIONS

In the summer of 2024, Alina Chan, a molecular biologist at the Broad Institute of MIT, published an essay in the *New York Times*.[15] That same Broad Institute of MIT hosts some of the most distinguished biologists in the world, such as cloning expert Rudolf Jaenisch. Chan explains in detail five key reasons why SARS2 did not originate as a natural spillover in a wet market, but rather, it came from some manipulation in a lab, most likely the lab in Wuhan. From my perspective, she gives a knockdown argument against the wet market theory.

It is certainly odd that an unknown, but dangerous new coronavirus emerged in a city that: (1) contained a major research institute that worked on bat viruses, and (2) that institute employed a scientist famous for her research on bats and their viruses, and (3) a bat-like virus emerged in a city far north of the usual habitats in caves of bats in China. It is also remarkable that, four years later, no consensus exists between either American federal agencies or famous science journalists about the lab-manipulation hypothesis, especially because SARS2 seems to exhibit evidence of being manipulated in a lab.

At best, the question remains unsettled. Congress continues to investigate EcoHealth and its funding with the Wuhan Institute for coronaviruses with novel traits that would make them more transmissible to bats (and possibly, to humans).[16] Certainly no one can prove that the new coronavirus did not emerge from something changed in a Wuhan lab, and a good deal of evidence points in that direction.

NOTES

1. Christopher Wray, "FBI director endorses theory COVID-19 virus may have leaked from Chinese lab," *Guardian*, February 28, 2023.

2. Jon Cohen, "CIA bribed its own COVID-19 origin team to reject lab-leak theory, anonymous whistleblower claims," *Science*, September 12, 2023.

3. Francis Sweeny, *Straight Talk MD* (podcast), https://podcasts.apple.com/us/podcast/straight-talk-md/id1060256849.

4. Donald McNeil Jr., *The Wisdom of Plagues: Lessons from 25 Years Covering Pandemics*, Simon & Schuster, 2024.

5. David Quammen, "The Ongoing Mystery of SARS-COV-2's Origin," *Breathless: The Scientific Race to Defeat a Deadly Virus*, Simon & Schuster, 2022, 315–40.

6. Nicholas Wade, "Where Did COVID Come From?" *Wall Street Journal*, January 29, 2024, A17. See also Nicolas Wade, "The Origin of COVID: Did People or Nature Open Pandora's Box at Wuhan?" *Bulletin of the Atomic Scientists*, May 5, 2021.

7. Peter Strobel, "Probe Targets Billing for COVID-19 Research," *Wall Street Journal*, December 23, 2023.

8. Jim Haslam, "Self-Spreading" Vaccines and the Origin of COVID-19 with Jim Haslam, *Straight Talk MD* (podcast), https://podcasts.apple.com/us/podcast/self-spreading-vaccines-and-the-origin-of-covid/id1060256849?i=1000629043548.

9. Ravi Iyer, *The Reaper's Dance: 1000 Days of COVID*, 2023, 102.

10. Debora MacKenzie, *COVID-19: The Pandemic That Never Should Have Happened and How to Stop the Next One*, Hachette, 2020, 19.

11. Andrew Rambout, quoted in Debora MacKenzie, Ibid.

12. Nicholas Wade, "Where Did COVID Come From?"

13. "Statement in support of the scientists, public health professionals, and medical professionals of China combatting COVID-19," *Lancet*, February 19, 2020, https://www.thelancet.com/journals/lancet/article/PIIS0140-6736(20)30418-9/fulltext.

14. Benjamin Mueller, "Republicans Step Up Attacks on Scientist at Heart of Lab Leak Theory," *New York Times*, May 1, 2024.

15. Alina Chan, "COVID Probably Started in a Lab," *New York Times*, June 9, 2024, SR6–7; Alina Chan and Matt Ridley, *Viral: The Search for the Origin of COVID-19*, HarperCollins, 2024.

16. Sheryl Gay Stolberg, Benjamin Mueller, and Carl Zimmer, "The Origins of the COVID Pandemic: What We Know and Don't Know," *New York Times*, March 17, 2023; Benjamin Mueller, "Republicans Step Up Attacks on Scientist at Heart of Lab Leak Theory," *New York Times*, May 1, 2024.

CHAPTER 7

Vaccines and Their Ethical Issues

I believe in vaccines. I was first in line to get the Covid vaccine, and as of the writing of this book, I have received eight shots (Pfizer). So far, and although I've surely been exposed to infected people, I've never gotten Covid.

I get the annual flu shot every year, and I haven't had a serious case of the flu in decades. (Like the Covid shots, flu shots don't provide sterilizing immunity; they just drastically lessen the effects of infection.) I am also vaccinated for RSV, shingles, and pneumonia each year. If I were younger, I would get the HPV-prevention shots.

I also don't like watching needles go in my body. I once almost fainted watching a needle enter my arm for a flu shot, and now I always look away. I know people like me who fear needles so much that they avoid all vaccines. For this reason, vaccines delivered by inhaling a mist would be great.

I mention my vaccine history at the beginning of this chapter because I want to emphasize that I believe in vaccines. Nevertheless, I understand that things can go wrong with them. To get informed consent from citizens about vaccines, two historical questions arise: (1) What historically went wrong with vaccines? (2) Did anything go wrong with the Covid vaccines? Vaccines also raise other ethical issues, such as equity in distribution among citizens, prioritizing essential workers, world-wide allocation, and governments suppressing misinformation about vaccines, but I discuss those issues in other places.

In general, not all anti-vaxxers are either crazy or stupid. Some have legitimate worries, especially if they tend to be hypersensitive to drugs and chemicals. Yet how can they trust authorities in public health if such authorities don't tell them the whole, complex truth?

HISTORICAL LAPSES IN DEVELOPING VACCINES

The creation and use of new vaccines against dangerous germs create many ethical issues, some not readily apparent. One important ethical question is: Should authorities disclose all past problems with vaccines?

On a personal note, when I wrote and published *Pandemic Bioethics*, several professionals in public health and medicine urged me to play down or ignore past problems with vaccines or any adverse reactions from Covid vaccines. I ignored their pleas, and I'm glad I did.

Four years after Covid first hit America hard, Apoorva Mandavilli, the veteran journalist who specialized in covering the pandemic, published in 2024 a front-page story in the *New York Sunday Times* about twenty Americans who had immediate, terrible reactions to a Covid vaccine, some of whom became disabled for years.[1]

In an accompanying opinion column, *New York Times* opinion columnist Ross Douthat explained how even this revelation would be filtered by both sides in America through preformed, political lenses.[2] Well, yes, of course, nothing will be reconstructed more in American politics today than the dangers or harmlessness of vaccines.

But let's go back in time to the beginning of vaccines. A quasi-vaccine, created by physician Edward Jenner in 1796, arguably stood on shaky ethical ground. Hearing and observing that women who milked cows and contracted cowpox fared better than others when infected with smallpox, Jenner reasoned that exposure to cowpox might protect those later infected with smallpox.

The idea was not original with Jenner. Long before him, African and Indian healers used variolation, where they injected bits of scabs of pus from mild cases of smallpox to lessen the effects of later smallpox. Variolation, also called inoculation, usually caused a mild case, but occasionally a variolated person became seriously sick or even died, so it could be dangerous. More on this later problem when we discuss the trolley problem with vaccinations.

Onesimus, an enslaved African, told Cotton Mather in 1716 that he had been given a mild dose of smallpox in Africa, could not get infected again, and that the practice had worked for a century in Africa. Mather urged British and Boston physicians to try it, but slaveholders saw it as a plot contrived by enslaved Africans to infect and kill their masters, so it never took hold.

Jenner used variolation, subcutaneously injecting bits of smallpox virus into James Phipps, a healthy eight-year-old who was the son of his servant-gardener, who, of course, could not consent and who was used as a Kantian means to the end of proving that variolation worked.[3]

Slowly evidence mounted that those who had been inoculated were more likely to survive during outbreaks of smallpox than those infected, so the practice spread throughout the Colonies. During the Revolutionary War, George Washington, who had survived smallpox as a teenager, used variolation on his army, even forcing some reluctant soldiers to accept it.

A hundred years later in France, Louis Pasteur had an opportunity to try his vaccine against rabies, a disease that was always fatal, but which, fortunately for him, after a rabid bite took weeks to develop. Using deadened, weakened forms of rabies virus present in rabbits, Pasteur produced a possible vaccine for humans.

On July 6, 1885, Pasteur got the opportunity he needed when a rabid dog bit Joseph Meister, a nine-year-old boy, many times. A physician friend injected Joseph thirteen times over ten days with doses that were progressively fresher, more virulent, and stronger, strengthening Joseph's immune system to fight the virus incubating inside him.

Pasteur's rabies vaccine worked, and like Jenner, Pasteur became a national and international celebrity. Utilitarians could justify the methods of both men, but Kantians could also justify Pasteur's approach.

Jumping to the 1950s in America, Jonas Salk created the first vaccine against polio, but he also inadvertently started the modern anti-vaccination movement. Salk used weakened, live virus in his vaccine, but he wrongly injected it first into his own children, either being confident that it would work or not caring about jeopardizing his children. Overall, his weakened virus worked well as a vaccine against polio.

Unfortunately, the Cutter Laboratories in California had sloppy controls, and they mistakenly produced vials with live polio virus rather than the weakened virus. As a result, of the millions of children who were vaccinated, about sixty-four thousand children contracted polio from a Cutter vaccine. Although polio is not serious in most children, the Cutter batch crippled 164 children with varying degrees of lifelong paralysis, and worse, it killed ten. A few of these children lived the rest of their lives in iron lungs, the predecessor of today's ventilators, and an awful symbol to Americans of the dangers of vaccination.

Swine flu vaccines also helped to inspire the anti-vaccine movement. In 1976, an outbreak of the swine flu at an American military base created fears of a devastating epidemic, like the Great Flu of 1918. President Gerald Ford quickly announced a plan to vaccinate all Americans. By the end of that year, nurses had vaccinated forty million (of two hundred million eligible) Americans, nominally a great achievement.

Fortunately, no epidemic developed, but the credibility of public health then suffered. Unfortunately, a small number of vaccinated Americans developed Guillain-Barré syndrome, a rare autoimmune disorder and lifelong condition wherein a subject's immune system overreacts to damage the peripheral nerves.[45] Of course, these people were worse off than if they had never been vaccinated.

In 2024, Abrysvo, a new vaccine for respiratory syncytial virus (RSV), was the only RSV vaccine approved for use by pregnant women and was not approved for kids. However, pharmacists got conflicting information and gave 128 women and twenty-five kids an alternative, unapproved vaccine.[6] Follow-up has started to see if any were injured by the mistakes.

Those encouraging everyone to vaccinate do not want to admit such lapses. Nevertheless, as one expert commented, vaccine manufacturing is an endeavor in which an almost-infinite combination of things must work perfectly, with variable raw materials and finicky microorganisms fueling key factors and needing to be grown in ideal conditions—in sum, "a science with established principles, but sometimes [which] is more idiosyncratic than art."[7]

As a result of such mistakes, in the early 1980s and as part of the National Childhood Vaccine Injury Act (NCVIA), the US government in 1986 created the National Vaccine Injury Compensation Program.[8] The specific cause for the NCVIA was the reluctance of parents to give children the standard DPT vaccine (against diphtheria, pertussis [whooping cough] and tetanus). This program is a no-fault alternative to lawsuits in courts, where claims are heard in a special vaccine court presided over by a special master of the US Court of Federal Claims.

The Risks of Covid Vaccines

As mentioned, one doctor in infectious diseases advised me not to mention any bad reactions to Covid vaccines. "They are one in a thousand, so anyone's chances of bad reactions are less than getting T-boned on their commute to work, but fear of such reactions will cause many not to get the shots, and as a result, to get very sick or die. Don't spread the fear!"

Such is the polarized state of all discussions in the United States about Covid vaccinations.

With the rollout of the Pfizer vaccine, two people in England and six in the United States had bad reactions, including a nurse in Alaska who suffered anaphylactic shock. In Boston, a physician had a strong allergic reaction to the Moderna vaccine.[9]

In Elmira, New York, the previously healthy twenty-four-year-old George Watts Jr. got a second shot of a Covid vaccine and later collapsed in his room. According to the medical examiner at the local hospital, myocarditis caused George's death, but the coroner's conclusion was controversial, although his diagnosis of myocarditis was not. As a retired forensic pathologist said, "The leap here is the conclusion that it is vaccine-related."[10]

For unknown reasons, the mRNA vaccines of Pfizer and Moderna can cause myocarditis in young men who get two shots.[11] Anti-vaxxer Robert F. Kennedy Jr. seized on this story, aided by George's father, who was convinced that the vaccine had caused the death of his son.

Overall, from late 2020 to mid-2022, there were 16,514 reported cases of myocarditis or pericarditis in people after getting Covid vaccines. After Americans received seven million dosages, at least 224 documented cases of myocarditis occurred. Across the world, and after m-RNA vaccinations for Covid, 128 known deaths from myocarditis occurred, primarily in males with a median age of twenty-five.[12]

It is also true that myocarditis is much more likely to develop after a Covid infection, and unvaccinated people are much more likely to get Covid, so the risk-benefit ratio for most people likely still favors vaccination.

In England, a thirty-two-year-old psychologist developed blood clots after the first dose of the AstraZeneca vaccine and died ten days later.[13] His death was described as related to blood-clotting syndrome, known as TTS, which had also occurred in Australia in two or three patients per one hundred thousand given the same vaccine. A British study also discovered that young women under the age of thirty were more likely to experience a deadly version of TTS, causing Britain to withdraw the vaccine in April 2021. Before the withdrawal, six young women who had gotten at least one dose of this vaccine died of cardiac-related problems. Because of such concerns, the AstraZeneca vaccine was never approved for use in America.

A study in October 2023 also found that the Pfizer and Moderna mRNA vaccines, when combined with a high-dose flu vaccine, increased the risk of stroke 20 to 35 percent, or three additional cases of stroke for every one hundred thousand people vaccinated.[14]

Despite these events, the overall risk of a severe adverse reaction from taking Covid vaccines for most people has been slight. Given the much greater risk of serious illness, hospitalization, or death from Covid, most people should get one of the vaccines. Nevertheless, there will always be some people who might have hyperimmune responses to Covid vaccines, and for them, the risk/benefit ratio differs.

GENERAL ETHICAL ISSUES OF USING NEW VACCINES

One of the things that evolutionary biologists and such have argued is that some people among us are hyperresponsive to dangers, whether socially, physically, or chemically.[15] They are the tribe's "canaries in the mine." Although being hyperresponsive is not good for the prairie-dog sentinel who yells when the wolf gets him, his cries can save the prairie-dog village.

With new drugs, some humans will always be hypersensitive. Even drugs and substances initially thought to be universally good, such as penicillin or peanuts, turn out to harm some people, even putting them into anaphylactic shock.

Thus, it is almost an axiom of vaccinology that any time a new vaccine is tested, or used on a large population, some individuals will be harmed, some will experience horrendous symptoms, and some may even die because of cytokine storms when their immune systems overreact to the new threat.

Thus, a problem exists anytime a new vaccine or drug is introduced. This problem occurred in the Philippines in 2016, when a small percentage of children suffered after getting the Dengvaxia vaccine for dengue fever. There, 830,000 children were vaccinated with Dengvaxia, made by a French drug company, Sanofi. Their parents were told that Dengvaxia would save their kids from getting dengue fever or from being hospitalized for it.

In truth, Dengvaxia did protect most children who had been previously exposed and who were likely to be exposed again, which was true of most of the 830,000 children who were vaccinated. However, parents were not told that for a small percentage of children who, by the age of eight, had never been exposed to dengue fever, Dengvaxia could make them worse off.[16]

What appears to have happened is that Dengvaxia made their immune systems hyperresponsive to exposure to the dengue virus, a phenomenon called "antibody-dependent immune enhancement."

Some such children were hospitalized, and some died, all of which was extensively reported by the Philippine media. Here was a perfect storm of apparent evil, right out of the movie/novel *The Constant Gardener*: a big pharmaceutical company from a developed country testing a dangerous vaccine on innocent children in a developing country, killing some.

In challenge studies of new vaccines for such viruses, antibody-dependent immune enhancement can occur. Challenge studies for Covid allowed volunteers to be injected with experimental vaccines and then be exposed to SARS2 to see if the vaccines worked.

But the ethical worry here was that a new vaccine would allow a quicker penetration of the coronavirus, making volunteers much sicker than they would have been if they had gotten SARS2 naturally.[17] So, should we tell volunteers that?

With the Dengvaxia vaccine, Kantians would argue that parents had the right to know the complex truth about the vaccine, even if telling the truth lessened vaccine uptake. Ideally, parents knew best whether their child had previously never been exposed to dengue fever, and hence, could be at risk from receiving the Dengvaxia vaccine. In retrospect, perhaps better, more truthful messaging would have been best overall, even on utilitarian grounds, to prevent the negative reaction that, in fact, occurred.

Another dilemma exists in testing any new vaccine. The people who need it most are also the people with the worst immune systems and the greatest burden from other medical problems. They are likely to be elderly patients suffering from several chronic and acute conditions.

Ethically, it seems difficult to justify trying out a new vaccine on them first, because placebos can't be used, and it might not work. On the other hand, if we don't try a new vaccine on some of them, how can we know how effective it is or even whether it is effective?

We also need to try new vaccines on some vulnerable, elderly patients for the good of the vast number of other vulnerable, elderly patients. But which few get sacrificed on the tracks? And who decides?

WHO MOST NEEDED COVID VACCINES?

How truthful should public-health leaders be if they want to create maximal acceptance of new vaccines? Some leaders believe that only simple statements should be used, such as "Vaccines work and save lives." These leaders resist saying, "Vaccines don't harm most people, they save the lives of others, but for a tiny number of people, they have serious bad effects." In other words, it seems permissible in government circles to tell less than the whole truth to the public to promote the greater good.

For example, it is well-known that the primary goal of vaccines is herd immunity, where most people in a society have either been vaccinated or gained "natural immunity" through infection. But does everyone need to be vaccinated for herd immunity to occur?

It seems not. As mentioned, the chances of a child dying from infection by Covid were less than a child's chances of dying from a mass shooting. On the other hand, the chances of a person older than the age of eighty-five dying of a Covid infection were 330 times greater than the odds of an eighteen-year-old dying from the virus.[18] Most college kids who became infected only had something like the flu, if that. So most healthy people under the age of twenty-five did not need to be vaccinated for a nation to achieve herd immunity.

But it's also true that eighteen-year-olds could carry the virus home to their elderly grandparents, who are at far greater risk of a poor outcome from a Covid infection, and on that basis, vaccinations were urged on them. Most people under the age of twenty-five could get Covid and easily survive, helping to create herd immunity with their subsequent "natural immunity" just as if they had received an RNA vaccine that tricked their immune systems into believing they had been infected.

With all that said, the public message might have been better stated like this: If you're over the age of sixty-five, if you've got a lot of medical problems, or if you're in a job with lots of daily, face-to-face contact, like a cashier in a grocery store, get vaccinated.

Another aspect of truth-in-public-health-messaging concerns truth-telling about what vaccines do for the recipient. It was widely, and falsely, believed by many Americans that getting vaccinated functioned like armor and prevented recipients from ever even getting infected (i.e., giving them sterilizing immunity). In truth, it only prevented worse-case illness from Covid because vaccines gave recipients a mild case of the virus, and hence, an immune boost.

Likewise, vaccines did not prevent those vaccinated from spreading SARS2, especially the highly transmissible Omicron variant. When vaccinated people spread this variant at Cape Cod in the summer of 2022, Americans felt betrayed by what they had previously understood from public health messaging, namely, that Covid vaccines could prevent recipients from passing on the virus to others or getting it again.

Conclusions

Vaccines for Covid or anything else are not perfect. Mistakes can be made while manufacturing them or injecting them, and they do carry risks of adverse events for a small number of people. Nevertheless, it's a shame that getting vaccinated has become so politicized and, in America, associated with resistance to officials in Washington, DC. But given the preceding political polarization that began occurring before Covid, and the mistakes in messaging made by officials during the Covid pandemic, in retrospect, it seems inevitable that such distrust of the Covid vaccine would occur.

In July 2024, a startling article in the *New England Journal of Medicine* lamented that when the official government vaccine committees pass on the safety of a new vaccine, they never authorize studies examining adverse events after the vaccine is given.[19]

Notes

1. Apoorva Mandavilli, "Could the COVID-19 Vaccines Have Caused Some People Harm?" *New York Times*, May 5, 2014, A1.

2. Ross Douthat, "How Politics Colors Our COVID Beliefs," *New York Times*, May 5, 2013, 3 (opinion section).

3. Proceedings of Baylor University Medical Center, January 2005; 18(1): 21–25.

4. https://www.who.int/bulletin/volumes/87/6/09-040609/en/.

5. Thomas Frieden, "The Three Key Hurdles for a Coronavirus Vaccine to Clear," *Wall Street Journal*, July 31, 2020. "Swine flu of 1976: lessons from the past," https://www.ncbi.nlm.nih.gov/pmc/articles/PMC2811391/.

6. Apoorva Mandavilli, "Errors Made in Who Got R.S.V. Vaccine," *New York Times*, February 15, 2024, A15.

7. Prashant Yadav of the Global Center for International Development, quoted by Elizabeth Weise and K. Weinbraub, "Pfizer Plants Across the Country," *USA Today*, February 9, 2021, D1.

8. National Vaccine Injury Compensation Program, https://www.hrsa.gov/vaccine-compensation/index.html.

9. Katherine Wu, "Boston Doctor Reports Serious Allergic Reaction after Getting Moderna's Shot," *New York Times*, December 25, 2020.

10. Stuart Thompson, "Out of a Family's Grief, a Polarizing Viewpoint," *New York Times*, December 17, 2023.

11. "Myocarditis after BNT162b2 Vaccination in Israeli Adolescents," *New England Journal of Medicine*, 387:19, November 10, 2022, 1816–18.

12. V. Jaiswa et al., "COVID-10 Vaccine-Associated Myocarditis: Analyis of the Suspected Cases Reported to the EudraVigilance and a Systematic Review of the Published Literature," *Int J Cardiol Heart Vasc*, December 2023; 49: 101280.

13. Michael Levenson, "U.K. Man's Death Tied to Reaction to Vaccine," *New York Times*, April 23, 2023.

14. Apoorva Mandavilli, "Two COVID Vaccines May Slightly Elevate Stroke Risk for Some," *New York Times*, October 26, 2023, A17.

15. E. O. Wilson, *Sociobiology: The New Synthesis* (25th Anniversary Edition), Harvard University Press, 2000, chapter 5, "Group Selection and Altruism," 106–30.

16. Lisa Rosenbaum, "Trolleyology and the Dengue Vaccine Dilemma," *New England Journal of Medicine*, July 26, 2018, vol. 379: 305–7.

17. This point was made in an interview with Professor Melissa Nolan, an "infectious disease expert" at the University of South Carolina on the BBC News, August 1, 2020.

18. Centers for Disease Control, "COVID-19 Mortality Update— United States, 2022," May 5, 2023.

19. D. Salmon et al., "Funding Postauthorization Vaccine Safety," *New England Journal of Medicine*, 391:2, July 11, 2024, 102–5.

CHAPTER 8

Truthful Messaging, Testing, and Public Trust

Veteran British science journalist Debora MacKenzie writes, "In any disease emergency, certainly in a pandemic, it is vitally important to tell everyone the whole truth—what we know and what we cannot know—and not hold back for fear of scaring people. That is a mistake that governments and other authorities make repeatedly with bad news stories like disease."[1]

Alas, that mistake was made in America.

Communications during Covid by officials in the Trump administration never had a chance of being truthful or trusted. As mentioned, on January 24, 2020, US deputy national security advisor Matthew Pottinger personally warned Donald Trump that the new coronavirus was very dangerous. Pottinger had served in China, and his wife worked at the CDC, so both had authoritative knowledge. As emphasized, on February 7, 2020, Trump told journalist Bob Woodward that the new coronavirus "goes through the air. That's always tougher than the touch. This is more deadly than flu. . . . This is deadly stuff."

Yet in public, Trump lied to Sean Hannity on Fox News on February 2, 2020, when he said, "We have it [the virus] totally under control. It's one person coming in from China, and we have it under control. It's going to be fine." On February 27, he misled Americans about the virus, substituting his hopes for what was likely: "One day—it's like a miracle—it will disappear."

The first scandal about truth-telling occurred on February 25, 2020, when the CDC's director for immunization and respiratory diseases Nancy Messonnier warned in public not only about imminent community spread of the coronavirus, but also that schools needed to make plans for teaching kids at home or apart with social distancing. The stock markets dropped 10 percent, and she was quickly forced to walk back her statement. She was never heard from regarding the virus again.

The reaction of the stock market so spooked Trump that he, and his financial advisors, decided that statements about SARS2 infections and Covid would henceforth be subservient to the needs of the financial markets.[2]

In 2002–2003, SARS1 hit South Korea, and as a result, when SARS2 broke out in Wuhan in 2020, South Korea had a plan. It developed a test almost overnight and successfully used aggressive surveillance, contact tracing, and quarantines to control the spread of the virus.

Yet according to Scott Gottlieb, the former head under Trump of the Food and Drug Administration (FDA), despite having an Office of Pandemic Preparedness, America lacked such testing and capabilities: "The US never developed a pandemic strategy that would be broadly relevant to a range of predictable and unexpected viral threats."[3]

Americans mistakenly assumed that leaders in the Trump administration in public health were medical professionals, not political appointees whose primary virtue in being chosen was their loyalty to Donald Trump.

Thus, on March 1, 2020, the CDC and US surgeon general Jerome Adams advised Americans not to wear masks in daily life to prevent the spread of the virus, advising them only to do so when near infected relatives.

Not only did American institutions make mistakes in leading and messaging, but so did the World Health Organization (WHO). Without sense, it criticized America for banning Chinese citizens from entering the United States. The same organization endorsed China's draconian lockdown of Wuhan's citizens. Thus, America did something that Taiwan, South Korea, and many Pacific Rim countries did, but when China barred any of the eleven million residents of Wuhan from leaving, something never done before in modern history, well, for the WHO, that was okay.

In retrospect, a bad moment for Anthony Fauci as a trusted public health servant occurred on February 1, 2020, when he assured a television host that SARS2 was not spreading in America, because if it were really spreading, "we would have an almost exponential spread of an infection, (one) which we are all looking out for."[4] Alas, we didn't have any tests when he said that, so we couldn't know.

Exactly what did occur was exponential infections, and more important, we didn't know then that such infections were asymptomatic for the first few days. Fauci also guessed wrong by extrapolating from the flu: "It would be unusual for an asymptomatic person to drive the epidemic in a respiratory disorder."[5] Yet that is exactly what happened.

In early 2020, American lacked tests for either the symptomatic or the asymptomatic SARS infection, and thus federal officials told the public false things. Why we didn't have a quick test, the way South Korea and Germany did, is a sad story.

Preparedness plans in public health assumed that a test would be developed quickly and that its results could be delivered quickly. These two things did not occur with testing for Covid. In a series of incredible mistakes, the United States did not use a test quickly created in Germany. Why is that an ethical issue? Because the delay in creating a useable test cost many people their lives, maybe hundreds of thousands.

In this regard, America did not learn from the needless deaths in France in the 1980s, when that country insisted on its own test for HIV, rather than using (and paying for) an American test, such that many Frenchmen needlessly died of AIDS.

Similarly, the CDC director Robert Redfield decided not to use the German test and insisted in late January 2020 that the CDC would create its own test and distribute it to the states. His reasons for this are still unclear, but it was a colossal mistake on many fronts: the Germans had a great test, already in use around the world. And it was likely caused by American hubris and narcissism.

From the very beginning of Covid in early 2020, no possibility existed of international cooperation: we weren't going to use a German test, nor were we going to share vaccines with any other countries. Meanwhile, thousands of Americans were returning on flights every day from Asia, even some from China.

The initial Covid test had three parts: two to test for the original strain of SARS2 from Wuhan and a third to test for variants of that original strain. Unfortunately, the person whom Redfield appointed to create the test for the CDC did not follow standard procedures for avoiding contamination with coronaviruses, which can be "sticky" in labs and negate results. As a result, the CDC's initial tests did not work, especially its third part.

At this point, the FDA could have granted emergency authorization for commercial labs to make their own tests, which such labs were eager to do, or for the CDC to just use the first two tests, but the FDA dithered, and the Trump administration, especially Alex Azar, head of the NIH, in a fit of jingoism, insisted on using the CDC's American test.[6]

Because we couldn't test for SARS2 versus strains of flu or the common cold—in other words, because we lacked a good test—no one then knew whether cases were actually spreading across the United States. As science writer Lawrence Wright described, for the CDC, this "testing fiasco" was "the lowest point in the history of a proud institution."[7]

In essence, the United States' refusal to use the German test cost America a month of testing. In retrospect, that set up America for many failures, especially defeating the possibility of prevention by contact tracing (see chapter 11).

If we had used the German test right away, we would have realized how quickly the virus had entered America and how quickly it was spreading. More important, such tests could have alerted us earlier to asymptomatic transmission. (Although most testing was for symptomatic people, if people started showing up in ERs who had previously been tested because they were near a positive case who, at the time of contact, was asymptomatic, we might have made the correct inference.)

MESSAGING DILEMMAS

I have some sympathy for officials in public health charged with protecting the public against dangerous germs. Whether it's contact tracing, isolation, quarantine, or all of the above, the introduction of any dangerous germ into the public sphere requires quick, decisive action. However, such actions often disrupt the lives of citizens, may spook the economy, and carry many collateral risks. As such, politicians will always be reluctant to believe that such actions are necessary.

Moreover, politicians may point to past overreactions, such as when President Gerald Ford had most of America vaccinated against the swine flu and then it petered out, leaving a small number of Americans with Guillain-Barré syndrome.

Perhaps the worst moment during the Covid pandemic for Anthony Fauci occurred on April 3, 2020, at a press conference called by President Trump, where the president reported that "Those in charge at the CDC now recommend that people wear masks" to prevent the spread of Covid, but he importantly then added, "This is *voluntary*, and I don't think I am going to be doing it."[8] Thus, on national television, Donald Trump pulled the rug out from under both Fauci and CDC director Robert Redfield.

On the other hand, if politicians and officials are too cautious and the germ spreads quickly, then at some point everyone realizes that something bad has entered the country, the public and starts to panic. At that point, containment efforts may be in vain, and officials will be criticized for not acting quickly enough.

Next, let's suppose officials convince politicians to act quickly, infected citizens are identified and isolated, and they successfully contain the spread. Then it may *appear* that there never was a real threat to the country or the economy. Heroes must work in private here.

Finally, given antigenic drifts in viruses, which causes them to constantly mutate and evolve, lots of small outbreaks occur all the time around the planet that do not gain traction, and hence, never pose any threat to humans. Officials can't cry "Wolf!" every time such a small outbreak occurs.

The classic trolley problem in ethics describes a spectator who can pull a switch on a runaway trolley car, which will hit ten people on its current track unless the spectator pulls the switch. If he does, though, it will hit one person on a different track. One way of thinking about the trolley problem in ethics is whether the agent will be left feeling bad about making a choice or doing nothing, as we saw when we discussed vaccines. The Dengvaxia vaccine in the Philippines illustrated a trolley problem: Should health officials allow a small number of kids to be harmed in order to save thousands of other kids?

Messaging about pandemics is a kind of trolley problem because it involves significant trade-offs: to be truthful about adverse reactions and mistakes in production and/or administration of vaccines and produce fewer citizens who take vaccines, or to underemphasize the dangers of a new germ to avoid a panic, but cause fewer citizens to take precautions. No matter what officials do, someone will criticize them, and some will feel bad about their decision.

Messaging, Again

Because American officials had no tests and thus couldn't detect community spread, they incorrectly assumed something false: that it was not occurring. As former FDA commissioner Scott Gottlieb wrote: "Government officials sometimes made the mistake of trying to answer every question [as if they knew the answer]. Sometimes when you lack the data, when you're confounded, the most reassuring message is to admit what you do not know. It builds trust, and building public trust is critical in a crisis."

For Gottlieb, public officials also made the mistake of telling the public "not to panic." When people hear that phrase, "There is no need to panic," the first thing many people will ask themselves is: "Should I panic?"[9]

Perhaps the worst example of an overstatement came when Anthony Fauci testified behind closed doors in 2024 that no hard evidence existed for the six-foot rule about social distancing, that it "sort of just appeared," and that "it was not based on any hard evidence."[10] People skeptical of the value of this distancing rule reacted angrily, wondering how a made-up rule could have come to so disrupt ordinary life. One irony here: the very approach that Fauci wanted to suppress, Focused Protection, also championed physical distancing to contain the spread.

Paul Offit, a physician of the FDA's Vaccine Advisory Committee and an author of many books and articles about vaccines who frequently appeared on television to discuss Covid, admits, "As the pandemic progressed, however, we found that we weren't always right, because our decisions were often based on incomplete information. At times we would give conflicting recommendations, and as a result, many Americans lost faith in the institutions and individuals responsible for protecting the public."[11]

After he resigned after four decades as head of the National Institute of Allergies and Infectious Diseases, upon reviewing America's efforts with Covid, Anthony Fauci concluded:

Something clearly went wrong. And I don't know exactly what it was. But the reason we know it went wrong is that we are the richest country in the world, and on a per-capita basis we've done worse than virtually all other countries. And there's no reason why a rich country like ours has to have 1.1 million deaths. Unacceptable.[12]

A remarkable confession from the man whom most Americans saw as our scientific leader during Covid, a man to whom, during the first year of the pandemic, many Americans listened.

HOW SHOULD GOOD LEADERS DISCUSS PUBLIC HEALTH DANGERS?

Let's admit the fact that when it comes to communicating with citizens, officials in public health during pandemics have difficult, even impossible jobs. Especially if they are political appointees, conflicting pressures constrict what they can truthfully say.

For them, the simplest strategy is always to use direct, absolute language and to push clear-cut rules, such as "Covid kills," or "Vaccinate everyone." This is an effective way to lead, and in the short run, it often gets desired results, but in the long run, truth wins out, and the truth is usually complex—more complex than simple, exceptionless rules.

Monica Gandhi argues that during Covid, fear-based messaging consumed public health rather than evidence-based messaging.[13] She theorizes that because Donald Trump minimized the dangers of Covid, public health and the mass media overemphasized the dangers, creating too many people fearful of too many things. Later, when kids and college students became infected and fared no worse than they would have with a bad case of the flu, people wondered why they had been so scared and started to distrust the messengers.

Fear about infection from contagious diseases has been used before. In the early twentieth century, the Syphilophobia Campaign attempted to frighten Americans about syphilis, portraying the disease as a rapidly fatal, incurable disease acquired by immoral behavior, with the only prevention being marriage among virgins who were faithful to each other for life. In the mid-1980s, when the actor Rock Hudson and a sex worker became infected with HIV, a magazine headline screamed, "NOW ANYONE CAN GET AIDS!"

Dr. Gandhi is probably correct that officials during the Covid pandemic had too many fear-based messages. The author remembers a mother married to a physician who refused to let her teenage sons leave their house, so fearful was she of their getting infected, and who made her physician-husband shower and wash his work clothes before entering the main part of their house. And he remembers family members who would not go to emergency rooms for fear of getting Covid.

Conclusions

In the long run, saying, "I don't know" can be effective. When true, it creates sustainable trust in public health.

Mistakes of messaging in public health, including not just mistakes about how to convey facts, but also whether such-and-such was a fact, caused massive reactions in state legislatures. At least thirty states passed laws forbidding county or state health officers from imposing measures restricting the liberties of citizens during future pandemics without explicit permission from the legislature.

In January 2023, after three years of listening to officials direct their lives about Covid, just half of Americans said they trusted American public health officials who had issued directives that affected their lives, a damning result.[14] Four years after Covid's start, New York's governor Kathy Hochul observed that many Americans distrusted government to protect them: "The pandemic pulled the rug from people—you were never quite as secure as you were. . . . I think it's just hard for people to feel good again."[15]

And one of the things they don't "feel good" about is leadership in public health. Although half trusted their personal physician to tell them the truth, about two-thirds lacked trust in either the CDC or the NIH to do the same.[16] Surely this lack of trust is one of the great losses caused by America's response to Covid.

In the summer of 2024, the great Turkish American columnist Zeynep Tufekci publicly lamented that how officials—including Anthony Fauci—communicated to the public about Covid destroyed public trust.[17] She is correct. And it's not just the many mistakes that were made and the backtracking, but *the way the mistakes were made*, with airs of absolute confidence.

On the shows that many Americans listen to, on radio and Fox News, a common theme is that Northeastern elites condescend to ordinary Americans and don't understand them. Whether it's about the harm of lockdowns on public schools and small businesses, or other hot-button issues like the inclusion of trans athletes in womens sports, many Americans feel that policies that affect them are being made by professional elites who are unlike them, and whom, consequently, they do not trust.

To end, again I ask the questions: Whose memory of this pandemic will prevail? Which kind of person will write it? Will it be written by politicians whitewashing their mistakes or critics who highlight those mistakes?

Notes

1. Debora MacKenzie, *COVID-19*, xix.
2. Gottlieb, 80.

3. Scott Gottlieb, *Uncontrolled Spread*, 4.

4. Gottlieb, 86.

5. Lawrence Wright, "The Plague Year," *New Yorker*, January 4 and 11, 2021, 30.

6. Ibid., 33.

7. Ibid., 34.

8. One reference to this is the interview with Anthony Fauci on *CBS Sunday Morning* that aired on June 16, 2024.

9. Gottlieb, 75–76.

10. Anthony Fauci, "Anthony Fauci 'Fesses Up," *Wall Street Journal*, January 11, 2024.

11. Paul Offit, "For the Next Pandemic," *National Geographic*, February 2024, 18.

12. David Wallace-Wells, "Interview with Anthony Fauci," *New York Times Magazine*, April 30, 2023, 39. Wallace-Well's reference for the per-capita figure is from *Our World in Data*, which reports 3,300 COVID deaths per million for the United States, 3,280 for the United Kingdom, and so on. Peru had 6,400 COVID deaths per million, but it is not a country America normally compares its health statistics against.

13. Monica Gandhi, *Endemic: A Post-Pandemic Playbook*, Mayo Clinic Press, 2023.

14. David Wallace-Wells, "Interview with Anthony Fauci," 8.

15. Lisa Lerer, "COVID Malaise Is Killing Trust in U.S. Politics," *New York Times*, March 25, 2024, A1.

16. Mary Van Rearden, "Survey reveals low trust in US public health agency information amid pandemic," CIDRAP: University of Minnesota, March 27, 2023, https://www.cidrap.umn.edu/covid-19/survey-reveals-low-trust-us-public-health-agency-information-amid-pandemic.

17. Zeynep Tufekci, "An Object Lesson on How to Destroy Public Trust," *New York Times*, June 9, 2024, SR6–7.

CHAPTER 9

Censoring False Messages about Covid and Vaccines

Readers might wonder why a chapter exists here devoted to whether talk about Covid should be censored by governments, and by extension, how governments should control information during future pandemics. My answer is first, that a significant moral issue emerged as to whether social media companies should champion or suppress views about Covid, and second, the moral issue encompassed whether government should make such companies suppress some views.

In the movie *Contagion*, Alan Krumwiede (played by Jude Law) hawks the fake cure "forsythia." Desperate patients listen to his podcasts and buy forsythia. In the movie, Krumwiede comes to a bad end, but similar fraudsters during Covid profited from such scams.

If readers embrace medical science, they may think, *Of course government should attack false claims about cures for diseases!* Social media should suppress misinformation about vaccines, and government should support such suppression. Falsehoods create vaccine hesitancy and foolish experiments with quack therapies, such as taking the horse dewormer ivermectin to treat Covid.

When questions arise about the role of government in suppressing views, things change. While some readers may have agreed with the Biden administration's attempts to suppress misinformation, once the principle is accepted that government has the right to suppress any information, we may be on a dark road. Consider what might have been suppressed had Donald Trump won the election over Biden.

No one questions whether governments have a role in providing correct facts, such as the calorie count on a package of oatmeal or whether meat has been inspected. But, of course, it's not that simple. The line between facts and values is not always clear, and such claims of "fact" can easily morph into claims about what people should do, the realm of values.

Moreover, most press releases contain an emotional spin, and this spin influences how the public receives the messages. But to generate trust, shouldn't such releases be as neutral as possible? Otherwise, is government overstepping its rightful role?

THE CENSORSHIP OF A FREE PRESS?

Regarding pandemics, to what lengths can state and federal governments go in banning views they don't like about vaccines and infectious diseases? Officials in the Biden administration attempted to restrict anti-vaccination rhetoric on the internet, especially on Facebook and similar social media platforms. Such actions caused an unusual legal case to be brought before the US Supreme Court in 2024 in *Murthy v. Missouri*. Individuals whose posts on social media about Covid had been censored were claiming their First Amendment rights to free speech had been violated.[1]

In its defense against the lawsuit, the federal government claimed it had sought only to *persuade* social media platforms to take down misleading posts about vaccinations, not *compel* such platforms to do so. However, former White House press secretary Jen Psaki did, in fact, threaten platforms that did not censor "vaccine misinformation," saying that they "could face legal consequences." Lower courts held that such threats went far beyond "persuasion."

This is interesting. The emerging field of social epistemology attempts to help citizens access the truth, in other words, to fact-check what they read on the internet. Much of what users see on Google, Facebook, Instagram, or TikTok is curated and mediated by algorithms, and certainly, some posts are outright banned, such as those that threaten to kill, rape, or bomb specific individuals or businesses.

France, Germany, Malaysia, Russia, and Singapore have all implemented laws against spreading fake news and health disinformation.[2] "Misinformation" can go very far: In England, the conservatives suspended Andrew Bridgen from their party in Parliament after he tweeted an article questioning the safety of vaccines and said a cardiologist had told him, "This is the biggest crime against humanity since the Holocaust."[3]

Given the hostility to Focused Protection during Covid, one wonders whether actual attempts were made to suppress it on the internet. Given the famous remark of Francis Collins about the Great Barrington Declaration ("There needs to a quick and devastating, published takedown of its premises"[4]), one can only suppose that efforts were made.

What about information that is misleading? Well, that is a problem, too. Consider the widespread slogan by the United Network for Organ Sharing that "Organ donation saves lives." This message is often wrapped in language extolling such donors as heroes. This campaign has been so successful that voluntary donations from living adults for kidneys surpassed those from cadavers in 2003.

Yet most donations of kidneys do not save a life; they merely get someone off dialysis, which has a high burden of symptoms, is prone to infections, and requires people to travel to dialysis clinics three times a week. Although kidney donations vastly *improve* the lives of recipients, most donations of kidneys don't *save* lives, even if UNOS implies otherwise.

Moreover, such donation is not risk-free. Some donors have been injured, and because the donation was voluntary, many of these injured donors have found themselves responsible for the subsequent medical bills—because their injuries were "self-inflicted."[5]

Similar benevolent deceptions surround calling brain-dead and anencephalic babies "heroic donors." Though not consenting donors, they are organ sources, nonetheless.

What about campaigns that say, "Vaccines save lives"? That is true, but it doesn't necessarily mean that the vaccine saves *your life*. For Covid-19, one study showed intentions to vaccinate at a country level were strongly influenced by trust in that nation's government. If that is so, how would censorship by governments increase trust?

It is also unproven that posts on social media create vaccine hesitancy. For example, in America, decades of mistrust of government medicine by African Americans, created by the Tuskegee Study, Henrietta Lacks, and the early use of Bruce Tucker for a heart transplant, created a legacy of mistrust among Black Americans about government-created vaccines. And when Melinda Gates suggested Black Americans should get vaccinated first as a form of reparations for historical injustice, her suggestion was widely interpreted as a ploy to turn African Americans into guinea pigs for an experimental vaccine.

In arguments about *Murthy v. Missouri*, lawyers for the Biden administration portrayed the federal government as merely suppressing "misinformation." They portrayed advocates of free speech and a free internet as shills for blatant falsehoods. They tried to take the high moral ground and portrayed their opponents as sliding around below in the mud of untested, goofy, "forsythia" scams. But the truth was more complex.

Conclusions

In June 2024, the US Supreme Court ruled six to three in favor of the Biden administration in *Murthy v. Missouri*, but they did so on the technicality that the suit brought by the state attorneys general lacked standing to claim harm on behalf of their citizens.[6] Moreover, the five individuals who had sued could only prove past harm from censorship, not future harm. Nevertheless, the Court left open the question as to whether specific individuals could similarly sue the federal government for the censorship of their posts, especially if they both had been targeted in the past and expected to be targeted in the future.

In conclusion, governments, at least the US government at present, should not be given the power to suppress alternative views about vaccines, the nature of Covid, or possible treatments. In the preceding chapters, we saw numerous instances in which high-ranking federal officials attempted to quash views they opposed, even when those views—such as Focused Protection— had solid evidence to support them. Second, American federal agencies, such as the CDC, the FDA, and the NIH, made numerous early mistakes about Covid, as did the WHO, and if they had been allowed to suppress criticisms or alternative views, how was the public supposed to learn about these mistakes? Additionally, what if more ominous things turn out to be true, such as that American virologists had some level of collaboration with the Wuhan lab and might have had some role in creating a vaccine in bats that jumped to humans? These questions aren't just for conspiracy buffs.

Finally, even if some readers think suppression of falsehoods is permissible—say, about the dangers of vaccines—the principle that governments should be allowed to suppress all dissenting views during pandemics is too dangerous to allow. Not all governments are blessed with great leaders, and sometimes bad ones get into power, so the system must have safeguards. Government officials who become accustomed to suppressing words and views during a pandemic may afterward be reluctant to give up that power. When it comes to power and politicians, the modern Cincinnatus is rare.

NOTES

1. Editorial, "Big Tech and Free Speech, Round Two," *Wall Street Journal*, March 18, 2024, A16.

2. "Should we criminalise those who spread misinformation about vaccines?" *British Medical Journal*, February 17, 2021.

3. Associated Press, "UK Conservatives suspend lawmaker for vaccine misinformation," January 11, 2023.

4. Editorial, "How Fauci and Collins Shut Down the COVID Debate," *Wall Street Journal*, December 21, 2021.

5. Gregory Pence, "Kant's Critique of Adult Organ Donation," in *The Elements of Bioethics*, McGraw-Hill, 2007.

6. Jed Rubenfeld, "Murthy Wounds, but Doesn't Kill, Free Speech on Social Media," *Wall Street Journal*, June 28, 2024, A 15.

CHAPTER 10

Abandoning the Dying and the Infirm

Nearly four years into the Covid pandemic, the *Wall Street Journal*'s Matthew Hennessey wrote, "To my mild shame, I largely did as I was told during the pandemic. I wore masks, got the shots, worked from home, worshipped online. I even stayed away from my father's house as he lay dying from cancer. I should have been there. I'll never get over that."[1]

I understand Hennessey's frustrations.

My Brethren grandparents, Charles and Vernie Burner, paid for my tuition at the College of William & Mary. As a child who spent my summers on their farm in the Shenandoah Valley, I bonded with Vernie, who supervised the kitchen, the big farmhouse, and the garden's produce. After a lifetime of hard toil, and later surviving the death of her husband, Vernie achieved her lifelong dream and bought a house in the small town of Woodstock, Virginia, off Main Street. There she lived happily for a decade during her eighties.

During graduate school and my first years at UAB, I tried to visit Vernie once a year, but some years were missing in this regard, and I have always felt guilty about not visiting more, especially considering our bond.

At one point, I learned that Vernie had only a few months to live and that my mother had moved her into a nursing home near Woodstock, so I then began to visit as often as possible. I am happy that time wasn't during the Covid pandemic, because if anyone had barred me from seeing her during those last months, I would have been very angry.

Yet that is exactly what happened to hundreds of thousands of American families who encountered the "No Visitors Allowed" rules at hospitals and nursing homes when they learned that Mom or Granddad was dying during the height of the Covid pandemic.

Those rules inflicted a *moral injury* on these families. They harmed elderly residents, hindering final messages to and from them and thus preventing emotional closure. They also inflicted moral injury on medical and nursing home staff, who were compelled to enforce policies they hated. Now, looking back, we need to ask: Were those good rules? Did they accomplish anything good?

One question concerns those whom the rules were supposed to be protecting. At the end of their lives, few people want to die alone. Death will come for all of us, and the best we can do is plan to meet it well, hopefully without too much pain and surrounded by the people who love us.

Bryanna Moore argued in the *Hastings Center Report* that the isolation techniques implemented during the pandemic destroyed traditional ways of dying with families.[2] Heartbreaking videos on cable news showed families tapping on windows outside nursing homes, waving to feeble, elderly grandparents inside. How sad.

Was this worth it? Enraged families in Alabama descended on the legislature and forced the passage of bills allowing family members—at their own risk—to be at the bedsides of their dying relatives. Seven other states passed similar bills.[3] Some reporters portrayed this as legislatures caving in to hysteria, but was it? One legal author argued that "There is no epidemiological or US federal or state requirement to prohibit visitation to (and thereby isolate) dying patients," and that the commonly imposed

"No Visitors Rule" adopted by hospitals and nursing homes failed to consider the moral damage caused by such rules.[4]

If an elderly relative is dying and if she gets Covid from visits by her family, the family is then responsible. For their part, who better to judge the risk than families? And if the relative is already dying, getting Covid obviously won't matter that much.

What if Granddad's kids got infected by saying goodbye to him in the nursing home? So what? There was almost no risk that younger kids would get very sick or die. And after being properly informed, families were surely the right ones to judge these risks, because they might have only one chance to talk to their mother or grandmother before she died.

Like the negative ramifications of thoughtless humanitarian aid, thoughtless Covid isolation hurt dying people. Such isolation made families violate their duties to dying relatives, leaving those families with guilt. It also made the staff feel horrible.

Deathbed visits may be the last chance for some relatives to seek forgiveness or closure with an elderly relative. Even though it's clearly a horrible thing to deny relatives these final encounters, this horror is difficult to quantify. It's not like counting the quantifiable number of infections or deaths. No one counts how many families couldn't say goodbye in person to their dying grandparents, but surely hundreds of thousands of families, maybe millions, were left feeling aggrieved in this way.

Here is how one clinical ethics consultant lamented the way patients during Covid had to die in isolation and how their family members also had to grieve in isolation:

People are being prevented from attending funerals, crying together, and holding each other in a time where being able to do so feels more essential than ever. We are grieving in isolation—something that comes close to an oxymoron in many cultures, where mourning is a shared, social practice. A spike in Covid-19-related prolonged and complicated grief is itself a potential public health crisis.[5]

If funeral services were held outside, or inside with social distancing, it's hard to understand why officials prohibited such services. And did prohibiting such services really prevent any infections?

Physicians found it hard to tell grown children they couldn't be there as their dad died. As one intensivist told me, "People were choosing to avoid care they needed because they knew they would have to go through it themselves without a support system. And in the cases where they were sick and had no choice, their families were not allowed to see them, or care for them."

Abandoning the Infirm in Nursing Homes

The harm caused by the abandonment of the sick and the dying are often described in official reports in technical language, masking the horrible reality. An investigation by the Associated Press discovered that for every two official deaths from Covid in nursing homes, another early death occurred from neglect, or "failure to thrive."[6]

And although the overall mortality rate for Covid was only 2 percent among Americans, Americans over the age of seventy-five had a hundred times the risk of death from a Covid infection as someone who was under thirty. Patients in nursing homes accounted for 40 percent of Covid deaths in America.[7]

There's more to the story here than just how relatives couldn't comfort dying seniors. There's a paradox here as to why so many Americans in nursing homes died in the first place because the lockdowns and isolation of clients inside nursing homes were supposed to *protect* those inside from infection. What happened?

As Covid spread to staff, who then had to isolate, and residents, who then had to be separated and given extra care, uninfected residents were often neglected and left alone by low-paid aides working long shifts with too many residents to care for. If relatives had known of such conditions and had been allowed inside, they could have helped with bathing, dressing, and group activities.

Focused Protection directs us to maximize the protection of those most vulnerable to serious illness and death. This should have included those who died early from isolation and neglect. If we had rigorously intervened for such people, fewer would have died. Almost certainly, relatives could have helped prevent deaths from failure to thrive.

Another factor causing deaths in nursing homes concerns the diversion of resources. Keeping millions of children at home meant millions of parents couldn't work, including as aides in nursing homes, creating shortages of staff. Requirements to isolate for two weeks after an infection caused these staff shortages, as well as low pay. In retrospect, spending less money keeping children out of school and more on extra staff for vulnerable seniors in nursing homes would have also saved lives.

CONCLUSIONS

Between 2018 and 2022, 2,800,000 to 3,300,000 Americans died each year, or roughly three million a year.[8] During the years of 2020, 2021, and 2022, Covid pushed these numbers up closer to 3,4000,000. Now we know that dying during those years often took place either in a hospital with only occasional contact with people in whole-body PPE suits—often on a ventilator or ECMO—or in an isolated room alone in a nursing home.

Most Americans who died during the three Covid years died without relatives at their bedside. We could have done better. Although extreme measures might have been justified in 2020, by 2022 they were unnecessary and imposed unnecessary burdens on families, staff, and the dying.

NOTES

1. Matthew Hennessey, "No COVID Compliance This Time Around," *Wall Street Journal*, August 23, 2023.

2. Bryanna Moore, "Dying during COVID," *Hastings Center Report*, June 29, 2020.

3. Stephanie Columbi, "States Pass Laws to Guarantee Rights to Visit Patients, Even During Pandemics," *National Public Radio*, March 27, 2022.

4. Mayan Sudai, "Not Dying Alone: The Need to Democratize Hospital Visitation Policies During COVID-19," *Medical Law Review*, September 13, 2021.

5. Bryanna Moore, "Dying during COVID."

6. Matt Sedensky and Bernard Condon, "Not just COVID: Nursing home neglect deaths surge in shadows," Associated Press, November 19, 2020.

7. Lawrence Wright, 43.

8. Centers for Disease Control, "Underlying Cause of Death, 2018–2022," April 30, 2024.

CHAPTER 11

The Failure of Contact Tracing

Many assumptions ground standard models in public health that supposedly can be used to slow the spread of infectious viruses. One of them is contacting people exposed to a virus and getting them to isolate to prevent the infection of others, even if they have no symptoms and might not even be infected.[1]

For Covid, that assumption about contact tracing proved decisively incorrect. In America, just about everything about contact tracing went wrong.

Consider certain current behaviors of Americans that would defeat the strategy of contact tracing: (1) They don't answer calls on their cell phones from strangers. (2) They don't reveal private information to strangers, even those who allege they work for the county health department, and this private information includes their in-person human contacts over the past few days. (3) They certainly don't tell strangers about their recent sexual encounters or use of drugs and alcohol, especially if they've done something illegal. (4) If they will lose their wages, they won't isolate, because they need to work to afford to pay for rent and food. (5) If they're unsure if they're infected, they still won't isolate. (6) They don't want anyone to monitor their activities and whereabouts, and certainly not for two weeks. (7) They don't feel they belong to mainstream America, and thus they aren't interested in sacrificing for that mainstream. (8) They don't trust officials to tell them "the truth and nothing but the truth" about Covid. (9) They believe the tests for Covid were often inaccurate. (10) They believe that the dangers of Covid were exaggerated. They knew teenagers who tested positive for Covid and weren't even sick. Why should they lose their wages for two weeks to prevent the spread of something that really was no big deal?

Considering these facts makes us realize why contact tracing didn't work for Covid—and why it never will work.

And don't tell me that contact tracers will knock on doors and be able to gather such information. Many Americans have the same distrust of strangers knocking on their doors as they do of strangers making cold calls.

Also, did I mention that one in three Americans owns a gun? And another 10 percent live with someone who does? It's going to take a brave contact tracer to get answers to sensitive questions from such people. And compliance with isolation for two weeks? Doubtful.

Americans value their privacy, and contact such as this by public health officials can feel intrusive and threatening. When asked how successful political polls were with cold calls over the phone for the *New York Times*/Sienna poll, it was revealed that only 2 percent of people who are cold-called will even answer and then respond truthfully.[2]

Contact tracing failed in New York City, where Mayor Bill deBlasio assured his constituents that contact tracing would slow the virus and protect them. Later investigations revealed that only 42 percent of infected New Yorkers who were called between June 1 and July 25, 2020, *provided even a single contact.*[3]

In the summer of 2020, it took ten to fourteen days to get results back from a Covid test. That delay defeated the motivation for self-quarantining, and thus it defeated contact tracing. Ten days or fourteen days after becoming infected, John Doe could have been in contact with a hundred people, who in turn could have been in contact with a thousand.

Contact tracing works only when privacy isn't protected. In China, virtually no privacy exists: smartphones and cameras track the movements of every citizen. Facial recognition has advanced to new heights in China, and cameras can recognize individual faces from a hundred feet away. Chinese people who jaywalk or abandon rented bicycles in the wrong place can be easily fined. If a Chinese citizen acquires enough demerits, he cannot fly or take a train. To travel anywhere, Chinese citizens in Wuhan during Covid had to download a color-oriented app on their phones that conversed with central computers. If they tried to travel outside the city of Wuhan, police checked their phones: it had to show the right color, or the person was not cleared to leave. South Korea and Iceland used similar phone apps, and citizens seemed fine with their governments knowing their every location and activity.

Such is not the case in America. For complex historical reasons, Americans value privacy, where the word itself often symbolizes personal liberty. For Americans, civil rights are limiting conditions on what the state can do to you, and such fundamental political rights predate the state.[4] Individuals in America do not exist for the state, but rather, it is the other way around. The state exists to protect the rights of individuals; individuals do not exist to protect the rights of the state.

Deep political divisions easily defeat contact tracing in some countries. If people are deeply divided, with one ethnic group pitted against another, or if they are deeply distrustful of the government, they are not going to cooperate with contact tracers. On the other hand, in countries whose citizens have high satisfaction and trust in the government, such as Iceland, Denmark, and New Zealand, the citizens cooperated. Also, if everyone already knows everyone else—as in Iceland—privacy is not a big concern.

CONCLUSION: THE FAILURE OF CONTACT TRACING IN AMERICA

All in all, the most basic assumption behind contact tracing is that the numbers of infected persons are relatively small and that by contacting possibly infected citizens and encouraging their good behavior, those numbers can be kept small. But what happened when the authorities were slow to start contact tracing and the number of infected was already five million? Given asymptomatic spread and many of the infected having no or mild symptoms, many of those infected could have had contact with many other people before learning of their infected status. Thus, in a country that had already allowed the widespread dissemination of the virus, contact tracing was largely ineffective.

Even as early as August 2020, six months into the Covid pandemic, many state and city leaders in America admitted that contact tracing had been a colossal failure. As the *New York Times* concluded then:

> *Contact tracing, a cornerstone of the public health arsenal to tamp down the coronavirus across the world, has largely failed in the United States; the virus' pervasiveness and major lags in testing have rendered the system almost pointless. In some regions, large swaths of the population have refused to participate or cannot even be located, further hampering health care workers.*[5]

By this time, one expert, David Lakey, the chief medical officer for the University of Texas system, quipped, "Contact tracing is [now] the wrong tool for the wrong job at the wrong time. Back when you had 10 cases in Texas, it might have been useful."[6] On the day this story was published, California already had 500,000 cases, and Texas had 442,000 cases.

Former *New York Times* science writer Donald McNeil Jr. concurred:

Asian governments quickly trained large cadres of contact-tracers. In Wuhan alone, 9,000 contact-tracers were working by mid-February [of 2020]. It was not until June that New York City had even 3,000. That program—intended to be a model for the United States—quickly fell into chaos. Few New Yorkers cooperated, and it was ultimately judged a failure.[7]

British science journalist Debora MacKenzie illustrated what it takes to make contact tracing work:

As it wrestled the COVID-19 pandemic to a halt in spring 2020, China eventually used a 6-person team for each case to track contacts. The European Centre for Disease Prevention and Control estimates it takes a hundred person-hours to track one case's contacts. . . . But you have to start early, before there are too many cases to track.[8]

A virus can quickly pass a threshold in a population where contact tracing can't work, not only because too many cases exist, but also because people truly may not know the person from whom they got it (as in asymptomatic transmission). And if patient zero is one of the occasional "super-spreaders," then things quickly become hopeless.

Where contact tracing worked, it was employed early and had these factors in play: (1) Citizens of the nation felt a *strong sense of community*, in other words, that "we're all in this together" in fighting the new germ. (2) Most citizens *trusted* their governments to enact measures that would minimize the harm of the new germ. (3) Most citizens *accepted the harms of invasions of privacy* and surveillance for the *greater benefit* of identifying infected people. (4) Most citizens *cooperated peacefully* with orders by government authorities to isolate until they were no longer contagious. Which countries did this? Mostly Scandinavian countries, where people are the happiest, trust their governments, and enjoy generous benefits.

The italicized words and phrases above are value words, words that reflect commonly accepted standards of morality—i.e., of how people should act and get along, how they should share burdens and benefits.

Alas, I do not think Americans in 2024 will accept those statements. If I am correct, then public health in America should abandon contact tracing as a first response to outbreaks of new germs. It needs a better model.

On January 2, 2024, a plane full of 367 passengers caught fire after landing and hitting a small plane on the runway of Haneda Airport in Japan. Unlike what would likely have happened in America, the Japanese passengers stayed calm, followed the directions of flight attendants, and resisted jumping ahead to open emergency doors or clogging the aisles to retrieve their overhead baggage. As passenger Aruto Iwama recalled, "Even though I heard screams, mostly people were calm and didn't stand up from their seats but kept sitting and waiting. That's why I think we were able to escape smoothly."[9]

Can anyone imagine a similar evacuation on an airplane filled with 367 Americans? Alas, I think not.

NOTES

1. Devi Sridhar, professor of public health and chair of global medicine, University of Edinburgh, interviewed on "Global Public Access with Fareed Zakaria," CNN, December 20, 2020.

2. "You Ask, We Answer: How the *Times*/Sienna Poll Is Conducted," *New York Times*, May 14, 2024.

3. Sara Otterman, "They Praised Contact Tracing Rollout: Workers Called It Chaos," *New York Times*, July 29, 2020.

4. I am indebted to Alasdair MacIntyre for this point. See his *A Short History of Ethics: A History of Moral Philosophy from the Homeric Age to the Twentieth Century*, Macmillan, 1966.

5. Jennifer Steinhauer and Abby Goodnough, "Contact Tracing Has Largely Failed in the U.S.," *New York Times*, August 1, 2020, A1.

6. Jennifer Steinhauer and Abby Goodnough, "Contact Tracing," A5.

7. Donald G. McNeil Jr. *The Wisdom of Plagues*, 42.

8. Deborah MacKenzie, *COVID-19*, 12.

9. Motoko Rich and Hisako Ueno, "As Flames Surged, Order Prevailed Inside a Japan Airlines Jet," *New York Times*, January 3, 2024, https://www.nytimes.com/2024/01/03/world/asia/japan-airlines-fire.html?searchResultPosition=4.

CHAPTER 12

Federal Largesse during Covid

Fearing tens of millions of deaths from Covid, China pursued a Zero Covid policy and enforced draconian lockdowns, but in doing so, it crashed its economy. The American economy did not falter like China's. Why? Largely because federal bailout packages prevented defaults on mortgages, evictions, or loss of businesses. Was that sound policy? Perhaps, but it also created problems.

The Trump administration, fearing an economic crash that would put millions out of work, came up with an idea. In March 2020, as stores and resorts closed everywhere, things looked bad. In a bold move, Congress passed the Coronavirus, Aid, Relief, and Economic Security (CARES) Act, also called the American Rescue Plan of 2021, infusing $2.2 trillion of borrowed money into the economy.

Congress also eased the financial burden of its citizens by extending direct tax credits to families for childcare; expanding eligibility for Medicaid, allowing millions of families to get medical treatment for their children at a minimal cost and allowing many parents to stay home and care for children, rather than paying for expensive daycare; allowing direct payments to households for self-employed people; passing the Paycheck Protection Program (PPP) for small employers, increased by $600 unemployment stipends; and sending $1,400 in stimulus money directly to most Americans. Through the Small Business Administration, it also lent money to small businesses and nonprofit organizations. It also encouraged states to increase unemployment benefits.

Although most Americans viewed it as dysfunctional in terms of helping people get through Covid, the US Congress did well. Moreover, if it intended to prevent a recession, it succeeded.

But not everything worked perfectly. After Hurricane Katrina hit in 2005, Congress created the "employer retention tax credit" (ERTC) to help employers keep workers on payrolls in New Orleans. As part of the CARES Act in 2020, Congress created a $55 billion fund for ERTCs to help employers survive Covid.[1]

Critics say government-aid programs have too much red tape and take too long to write checks during emergencies. In contrast, when hurricanes or tornadoes hit areas, private insurance companies dispatch agents to customers in these areas and write checks on the spot.

Anticipating criticisms, the US government did not ask many questions or require much proof for employers to get ERTCs during the Covid pandemic. ERTCs in 2020 had a cap of $5,000 per employee, but when Congress extended ERTCs in 2021, it upped the amount to $7,000 per employee per quarter, or $28,000 a year.

However, even if businesses had received a loan to get paychecks flowing under the Paycheck Protection Plan, they also applied for ERTCs. Indeed, any business started during 2021 with employees could claim the tax credits, and even claim them retrospectively until April 2025.

But this loophole ended badly. According to a review in the *Wall Street Journal*, "The ERTC didn't help businesses survive or reduce layoffs. Only after the lockdowns ended did millions of employers apply to exploit the credit. Now the IRS is scrambling to down the open bar."[2]

I first became aware of a potential problem in early 2024, when I heard a questionable ad on a radio station, urging employers to file for ERTCs "even if you don't think you are eligible." The announcer gushed excitedly that there was "billions of Covid relief money allocated by the government, just for the asking," and correctly stated that "you can still claim your money years later, long after Covid has passed."

So started a wave of fraud created by sleazy companies that the Internal Revenue Service has struggled to control. Companies advertising on the radio could collect 20 percent of future payments for helping employers file for ERTCs. There was even an inmate inside a California prison who was able to defraud the US government of $550 million in ERTC money, filing hundreds of payroll tax returns that claimed ERTC benefits for ineligible and nonexistent companies.[3]

All an employer had to show was that revenue had declined during the Covid years—when everyone was staying home—easy to do for a typical restaurant, bar, or resort. Also, when employers paid nonworking employees through ERTC, they did not need to pay the normal taxes for workers for Medicare and Social Security. Thus, employers got tremendous benefits by filing for ERTCs.

Several companies emerged to help employers claim up to $26,000 per employee in tax credits, among them ERTC Specialists of Orem, Utah, which claimed to have helped sixty-five thousand employers claim credits, and by the end of the ERTC program, it had processed $10 billion in ERTC refunds.[4]

ERTCs worked well in 2020 and 2021, but by 2022, con artists had created many problems. By early 2024, when I heard the radio ad for it, everyone agreed that fraud was rampant.

Overall, the CARES act was one of the boldest economic-stimulus plans in US history. Given the pressures present during the Covid pandemic, it is understandable that it was not carefully planned, an actual shot in the dark. Some economists described it as "helicopter money," meaning that it wasn't that different from flying a helicopter over a city and dropping money on citizens below.[5]

Indeed, the federal government rained down so much money on states and businesses that some money was never spent. Between March 2020 and March 2021, Congress allocated $4.6 trillion to help Americans and businesses get through Covid, yet by March 2023, $444 billion of that total sat unspent.[6]

An interesting wrinkle in this federal largesse concerns death benefits. Part of the Covid Relief Act paid families and funeral homes for unexpected deaths from Covid, as much as nine thousand dollars per person or thirty-five thousand dollars per family. By 2023, the government had paid almost three billion dollars for Covid deaths. If doctors listed "Covid" on a death certificate, families got the benefit, and so even if cancer or heart disease had really killed the relative and testing positive for Covid was incidental, families pressured doctors to list the deaths as being from Covid.[7] Of course, this inflated the counts of American Covid deaths.

Despite the fraud in ERTCs, along with countless other errors and wastes of federal money, America did prevent a major recession. After the bundled mortgage fiasco in 2007–2008 almost caused the banking system to collapse, the Federal Reserve averted a similar disaster with other sensational moves, as detailed by Michael Lewis's (2021) *The Big Short*.

Eventually, however, the ERTC program became an embarrassment. Originally planned to cost $55 billion, as of the start of 2024, it had cost $230 billion.[8] Because employers can back-file from 2024 for claims from 2020, one analyst thinks the ERTC program may ultimately cost $550 billion.[9]

The CARES Act allowed the Small Business Administration to make four million loans to small businesses during the Covid pandemic, loaning in total about $390 billion. Unlike the forgivable loans of the Paycheck Protection Program, these loans, with a thirty-year fixed interest rate of 3.75 percent, had to be repaid with interest. By March 2024, one million of these loans were in default.[10] This is understandable because recipients of government loans (including students) tend to regard them as gifts, not as real loans that must be paid back.

One problem with paying back such loans is that many small businesses failed, such as Dan Presti's bar and restaurant on Staten Island, and thus they could not make the payments. A mattress company in Nashville in 2020 borrowed $450,000, but after people stopped buying mattresses during Covid, it failed, with no money left to pay its creditors.

Although the owners of such failed businesses can apply for hardship deferrals, by March 2024, the Small Business Administration had already written off 20 percent of its $390 billion portfolio due to causes such as death of borrowers, fraud, or bankruptcy. The Office of Inspector General found that one-third of borrowers never intended to repay these loans, with evidence of fraud that indicated the loans would probably never be repaid.[11]

Congresspeople criticized the loans as giveaways, and after only three hundred thousand of four million loans had been repaid, they pressed the SBA to collect on the 3.7 million dollars of outstanding loans.

One lesson that small businesses learned here: the US government doesn't need a judge to allow it to collect debts. For people who are self-employed or own a business, this means the government can garnish their tax refunds or Social Security payments, the same way it can to collect on student loans.

BONANZAS FOR PHARMACEUTICAL COMPANIES

Of course, the major beneficiaries of the tsunami of Covid money were the pharmaceutical companies. The Trump administration threw billions at every plausible, and some not-so-plausible, company that claimed it could create a safe Covid vaccine. It even hedged by purchasing ten million doses of the AstraZeneca vaccine, even though that vaccine was never used in America and simply sat in warehouses.[12]

Government recommendations for Covid booster shots, and for future annual booster shots against Covid, meant that huge profits for these companies will continue, especially from sales to the US government of its vaccine, along with antiviral pills. In 2022, Pfizer became the first pharmaceutical company to make $100 billion in annual sales, and Moderna saw the value of its shares then increase by 1,000 percent.[13]

One less-obvious thing that Covid did for Big Pharma was to provide a PR bonanza. Between 2006 and 2012, pharmaceutical companies had been the villains by flooding America with *seventy-six billion* opioid pills.[14] Covid made Americans entirely forget about how this happened, even though a hundred thousand Americans still died of overdoses every year.

In retrospect, Operation Warp Speed (meant to accelerate the production of an effective Covid vaccine) did waste billions, but it also succeeded. And despite funding their research with public money, it also gave proprietary rights over vaccines to Pfizer and Moderna. Alas, that was both part of the attraction for these companies and the way most research on drugs and devices works in America.

CONCLUSIONS

Everett Dirksen, US senator from 1959 to 1969, once reportedly said, "A billion here, a billion there, and pretty soon you're talking real money." For Covid relief, the US government allocated "a trillion here and a trillion there," and ultimately, it did spend real money.

It was inevitable that some fraud would occur in programs designed to quickly inject cash into the economy and prevent business failures. Trillions of dollars went to big businesses, small businesses, childcare centers, laid-off workers, and struggling parents, most of which helped to save the American economy, allowing the United States to emerge from Covid economically stronger than China and many European countries.

Little noticed or appreciated, Congress also fixed gaps in American infrastructure in broadband, transportation, health care, science, and technology: $9 billion for vaccine distribution, $218 billion for improved transportation, $54 billion for scientific research, $65 billion for broadband to connect rural schools and communities, and $716 billion for states to modernize hospitals, schools, and clinics.[15]

NOTES

1. Richard Rubin, "COVID Tax Credit Became Big Mess," *Wall Street Journal*, December 26, 2023.

2. Editorial, "The Biggest COVID Scam," *Wall Street Journal*, December 28, 2023, A18.

3. "ICYMI: California Inmate's ERTC Fraud Scheme Underlines Need for Repeal," March 21, 2024, https://gop-waysandmeans.house.gov/icymi-california-inmates-ertc-fraud-scheme-underlines-need-for-repeal/.

4. Ruth Simon, "Pandemic Tax Break Sparks Suit over Fees," *Wall Street Journal*, 2024.

5. The COVID Crisis Group, *Lessons from the COVID War*, 123.

6. Joel Zinberg, "The COVID Slush Fund," *Wall Street Journal*, May 7, 2023.

7. Leslie Bienen and Margery Smelkinson, "The Vicious Circle of COVID Boondoggles and Bad Data," *Wall Street Journal*, January 26, 2023.

8. Editorial, "The Biggest COVID Scam," *Wall Street Journal*, December 28, 2023, A18.

9. Andrew Moylan, "A $550 Billion Pandemic Relief Scam," *Wall Street Journal*, January 25, 2024, A13.

10. Ruth Simon, "U.S. Seeks to Collect Billions in COVID Loans," *Wall Street Journal*, March 7, 2024, A1–2.

11. Arthur M. Diamond, "The SBA and My Fake COVID Potato Farm," *Wall Street Journal*, March 20, 2024, A13.

12. Elizabeth Cohen, "Government vaccine advisers say they don't foresee AstraZeneca vaccine being used in the US," CNN Health, April 2, 2021, https://www.cnn.com/2021/04/09/health/vaccine-advisers-astrazeneca-us/index.html.

13. Allysia Finley, "The COVID Vaccine Windfall Turns for Pfizer and Moderna," *Wall Street Journal*, November 20, 2023.

14. Scott Higham, Sar I. Horwitz, and Steven Rich, "76 Billion Opioid Pills: Newly Released Federal Data Unmasks the Epidemic," *Washington Post*, July 16, 2019. See also Gregory Pence, *Overcoming Addiction: Seven Imperfect Solutions and the End of America's Greatest Epidemic*, Rowman & Littlefield, 2020.

15. Charley Locke, "Where It Went: How the unprecedented flood of federal relief money is a boon to science and technology," *New York Times Magazine*, November 28, 2021, 41.

CHAPTER 13

Failures of International Cooperation

The World Health Organization (WHO) created EWARS, its Early Warning, Alert, and Response System.[1] It also created "EWARS in a Box," a system of applications for cell phones, landlines, and various communication platforms, allowing labs to quickly analyze new infections.

Outbreaks of Ebola or cholera seem perfect for EWARS, as no country would want such diseases to spread and most need help to curtailing the spread. Ideally, when a bad germ emerges and seems to be spreading, the relevant nation will alert EWARS, and EWARS will coordinate efforts to stop the spread. At least, that's the theory.

Of course, the EWARS system has flaws. If a new infection is self-limiting in, say, Zambia, an early notification to EWARS will harm Zambian tourism, and its international businesses, all for nothing.

Second, if Zambia cooperates with EWARS and reports an outbreak, some will blame it for the outbreak. Unfortunately, a long history of blaming exists, as does an equally long history of countries trying to escape blame, dating to 1918, when the American media successfully called an outbreak in Kansas "the Spanish flu."[2]

In the first year of COVID, neither the CDC nor the WHO had learned to avoid the use of labels that encouraged blame. Authorities first called variants of SARS2 "the English variant," "the Indian variant," and "the South African variant." With each label came a new fear of traveling to that particular country of origin. Donald Trump worsened the blame by calling SARS2 "the Kung flu virus" and "the Wuhan virus." China immediately understood that the world would blame it, so it blocked researchers from coming to Wuhan to discover how the outbreak had occurred.

Therefore, because of potential harm to the economy of the country of origin and the likelihood of blame for a new germ, countries will be unlikely to cooperate with EWARS, so we cannot depend on it for an early warning.

THE JENNER INSTITUTE

As described previously, in 1796, the English physician and scientist Edward Jenner created the first vaccine for smallpox, for which he became an international celebrity. The Jenner Institute was named for him in 2005; it is a nonprofit organization at Oxford University whose goal is to create cheap vaccines for the world's poor.

With SARS2, and in partnership with AstraZeneca, it hoped to vaccinate essential workers in all developing countries.[3] In doing so, it practiced *vaccine globalism*. In 2020, it successfully developed the Oxford-AstraZeneca vaccine using a modified adenovirus found in chimpanzees.

However, pharmaceutical companies Pfizer and Moderna created better vaccines, ones that mimicked spike proteins on the surface of the SARS2 virus. These vaccines used messenger DNA, or mRNA, to jump-start a person's own immune system to create antibodies to neutralize SARS2, blocking it from hijacking normal cells and replicating.

The first dosage of the mRNA vaccines primed the recipients' immune systems to fight SARS2, and the second dosage built it up more, such that when the real SARS2 virus came along, it could be weakened. The great benefit of these mRNA vaccines was that neither used weakened or dead coronavirus to build up immunity, so both created fewer allergic reactions than traditional vaccines would have caused. Moreover, mRNA vaccines did not need to be grown in chicken eggs, a medium that causes allergic reactions in some people.

With the first two million initial doses of AstraZeneca vaccinations, about three hundred people suffered anaphylactic reactions, and then, after over thirty-four million people had received AstraZeneca vaccinations, 222 people developed a rare blood-clotting disorder.[4] These reactions were about the same as adverse reactions from most previous vaccines that were derived from animals and grown in chicken eggs, but the results indirectly showed the superiority of the mRNA vaccines.

Neither the Jenner Institute nor AstraZeneca profited from making and distributing their vaccine. AstraZeneca made two billion doses at a cost of a few dollars per dosage.[5] Even after the US government gave Pfizer and Moderna billions to make their vaccines, each charged the government about twenty dollars for a shot of their vaccines to Americans (the commercial price for others was closer to one hundred dollars a shot).

When the Pfizer and Modern RNA vaccines proved safer to use, Western countries chose them, leaving the undeveloped countries to use the AstraZeneca vaccine. As of January 2022, approximately thirty-four million people worldwide have received 2.5 billion doses of the AstraZeneca vaccine.[6]

THE GLOBAL ALLIANCE FOR VACCINES AND IMMUNIZATIONS (GAVI)

In the spirit of the Jenner Institute, the Global Alliance for Vaccines and Immunizations (GAVI) brought together the

WHO, the World Bank, the Gates Foundation, and private donors to vaccinate medical and essential workers around the world.[7] AstraZeneca's CEO repeatedly promised that, with its partnership with the Jenner Institute, it would not profit from its vaccine.[8]

GAVI originally hoped to distribute two billion doses, and it endorsed a program called Covid Vaccines Global Access (COVAXX).[9] Over 160 nations agreed to cooperate this way, but not the United States.[10]

As 2020 ended, and as COVAXX had only secured a half billion dosages of various vaccines for the four billion people in developing countries, it looked as though developing nations would not get enough vaccines.[11] As of September 8, 2021, COVAXX had only distributed 240 million vaccine doses in 139 countries, well short of its goal of two billion doses.[12] Because Moderna priced its two-dose vaccine at sixty-four to seventy-four dollars and Pfizer/NBiotech at thirty-nine dollars for the same, COVAXX could only afford and distribute the AstraZeneca vaccine, priced at $3.50 a dose.[13]

Unfortunately, the manufacture of the AstraZeneca vaccine depended on the Serum Institute of India, a gigantic pharmaceutical company with a reputation for producing generic drugs of high quality. When the Delta variant hit India hard in 2021, the government of Premier Narendra Modi prevented four hundred million dosages from this Institute from leaving India, keeping them at home to vaccinate Indians.[14]

As David Heymann, a fellow at London's Chatham House Global Health program, explained, "Most countries are going to be politically obliged to make sure it [the successful vaccine] goes to their own people if it's being produced and manufactured in their own country."[15] Vaccine nationalism explains why the United States bought Pfizer's vaccine and gave Moderna two billion dollars for first rights to its use.[16]

The nationalistic vaccine grab by India doomed GAVI's and COVAXX's efforts. Moreover, India forced poor countries to negotiate for vaccines from Pfizer and Moderna on their own rather than relying on COVAXX.

COVAXX had its critics. Most of its vaccines arrived too late to flatten the curve in developing countries.[17] It also allowed people in those countries who could pay to jump to the front of the queue.

Another serious blow to GAVI was that it had to order vaccines from manufacturers late, after many governments had secured dosages for their citizens from the same manufacturers. COVAXX also gave mRNA vaccine manufacturers thirteen billion dollars in advance for shots, but then the demand worldwide plummeted as only milder Omicron variants spread. The final indignity was that Pfizer and Moderna kept $1.4 billion of Gavi's money for canceled shots, which they were legally entitled to keep, but which was a public relations nightmare for GAVI.[18]

Globally, vaccine hoarding by America, Canada, and Japan horrified poor countries. At one time, Canada and America had enough vaccines to vaccinate each citizen six times. Even more astonishing, when half of Americans refused to get vaccinated, America (as well as Canada and Japan) still kept the unused vaccines instead of giving them to poor countries, and then the stored vaccines eventually expired.

Critics wondered why the public should have to allow Big Pharma to profit from vaccines that it had financed, but that is true for many devices and drugs. For most things funded for discovery and research by the NIH, drug companies are still allowed to patent, sell, and profit from their discoveries.

Conclusions

In 2021, Dr. Michael J. Ryan, director of health emergencies for the WHO, chided that giving booster shots to already-vaccinated

Americans was like "handing out extra life jackets to people who already have life jackets while leaving others to drown."[19]

After delivering nearly eighty-four million doses of vaccines to 146 countries, and probably preventing 2.7 million deaths in developing countries, COVAXX ceased to exist on December 31, 2023.[20] After ceasing the production of its vaccine, on May 8, 2024, AstraZeneca pulled its vaccine from global markets, citing low demand.

NOTES

1. WHO, https://www.who.int/emergencies/surveillance/early-warning-alert-and-response-system-ewars.

2. John Barry, *The Great Influenza: The Story of the Deadliest Pandemic in History*, Viking, 2004.

3. "Should Oxford-AstraZeneca's Progress Worry Moderna?" *Forbes*, July 22, 2020.

4. "AstraZeneca's COVID-19 vaccine: EMA finds possible link to very rare cases of unusual blood clots with low platelets," *European Medicines Agency (EMA) press release*, April 7, 2021, archived from the original, from May 20, 2021, retrieved April 9, 2021. Text was copied from this source, which is © European Medicines Agency. Reproduction is authorized provided the source is acknowledged.

5. Associated Press, "AstraZeneca: No profits from COVID Vaccine," *Tuscaloosa News*, July 31, 2020. Even folks associated with the Oxford vaccine are not angels, and some would profit from a successful vaccine, including Oxford University itself, the two lead scientists, and a private investment firm providing some of the startup capital. Jenny Strasberg, "Private Investors Stand Ready to Profit from Oxford Vaccine," *Wall Street Journal*, August 3, 2020.

6. "One year anniversary of UK deploying Oxford-AstraZeneca vaccine," gov.uk, January 4, 2022.

7. WHO, https://www.who.int/initiatives/act-accelerator/covax.

8. Associated Press, "AstraZeneca: No profits from COVID Vaccine," *Tuscaloosa News*, July 31, 2020.

9. Adam Taylor, "Why Vaccine Nationalism Is Winning," *Washington Post*, September 3, 2020.

10. Richard Engel story on GAVI, *NBC News*, July 31, 2020.

11. Saheed Shah, "Developing Nations Press Vaccine Access," *Wall Street Journal*, November 18, 2020, A8.

12. Jamie Ducharme, "COVAX Was a Great Idea, but Is Now 500 Million Doses Short of Its Vaccine Distribution Goals. What Exactly Went Wrong?" *TIME*, September 9, 2021.

13. Peter Loftus, "Drugmakers Start to Signal Prices for COVID-19 Vaccines," *Wall Street Journal*, August 5, 2020.

14. Stephanie Nolen, "Covaxx May End Its Effort to Vaccinate Poor Nations," *New York Times*, December 8, 2022, A11.

15. Peter Loftus and Drew Hinshaw, "Countries Vie to Get First Dibs on Vaccine," *Wall Street Journal*.

16. Rick Bright, PhD, the former director of BARDA, was transferred to a meaningless job by Trump for telling the truth about the lack of readiness in the United States to fight the virus. Peter Loftus and Drew Hinshaw, "Countries Vie to Get First Dibs on Vaccine," *Wall Street Journal*.

17. "COVAX Ends, COVID-19 Vaccinations Become Regular Immunization," *Mirage*, https://www.miragenews.com/covax-ends-covid-19-vaccinations-become-regular-1147009/#google_vignette.

18. Stephanie Nolen and Rebecca Robins, "Coronavirus Vaccine Makers Kept $1.4 Billion for Canceled Shots," *New York Times*, February 2, 2023, A9.

19. Quoted by Donald McNeil Jr., *The Wisdom of Plagues: Lessons from 25 Years Covering Pandemics*, Simon & Schuster, 2024, 193.

20. WHO, https://www.who.int/initiatives/act-accelerator/covax.

Rethinking Vaccine Mandates

In August 2021, President Biden ordered all federal employees, including the employees of the Veterans Administration, to get the Covid vaccine or undergo strict testing and masking protocols. California's governor Gavin Newsom and New York's governor Andrew Cuomo did the same for their state employees. In 2021, secretary of defense Lloyd Austin required all members of the US Armed Services to get vaccinated, achieving 98 percent compliance. Nevertheless, these actions were taken when the FDA had only given Covid vaccines "emergency use authorization," not "full approval."

ADVOCATES FOR VACCINE MANDATES

If the "greater good" justifies the mandatory vaccination of children for them to attend public schools, could it also justify the mandatory vaccination of adults? Three professors at Case Western Reserve University argued that national herd immunity could only be achieved this way.[1]

So, how to enforce such mandatory vaccination? First, the professors proposed denying religious objections to vaccination, stating that "the major religions do not oppose vaccinations." They also would reject any personal objections to vaccinations, because, they said, such objections "violate the social contract."

Second, to get high vaccination rates, they argued that governments should refuse tax credits and some government benefits to vaccine refusers. Health insurers should charge refusers higher premiums. Schools should refuse to teach unvaccinated children. And airlines, trains, and buses should not allow unvaccinated citizens to travel.

What about citizens who needed to travel or work in different places? These professors propose a national vaccine "certification card," with an expiration date, for everyone in the country, whether "here legally or not." Although the authors admitted their proposals were draconian, they argued that the alternative, a sustained pandemic, had unacceptable costs.

Both Anthony Fauci and science writer Donald McNeil Jr. argued that ordering and enforcing vaccine mandates would save lives. Both Fauci and McNeil thought the government should have gone much further in New York City and Washington, DC than making it difficult to get into good restaurants. Instead, they believed such large cities should have followed Asian countries, entirely banning the unvaccinated from buses, subways, airplanes, ferries, and grocery stores. McNeil thought the Biden administration "lacked the courage" to do so.

But was it simply a matter of "lacking courage" to do the right thing, or did doubt exist about what exactly the nature of the right thing was to do?

Is mass, mandatory vaccination even possible in America? In this country, many Americans resisted something as minor as wearing a mask, and for many others, invasion by the state of their body in the form of an injection/vaccine is an ethical red line that should not be crossed.

In 1902, the city of Cambridge, Massachusetts, made vaccination against smallpox mandatory for its citizens, a law that even survived a challenge in the US Supreme Court. But how far did Cambridge go to secure such vaccinations? A hundred years ago, officials went door to door requesting proof of vaccination, and if someone didn't have it, they were vaccinated on the spot. Could such a scenario occur today in America for the Covid vaccine? Is it relevant that America today is a country where 30 to 40 percent of households have guns? Let's just say I wouldn't want to be the public health officer trying to enforce such a mandate by going door to door with a vaccination syringe in hand, ready to administer.

CRITIQUE OF VACCINE MANDATES

In democracies, mandatory vaccination policies rub against individual rights to control one's own life and body. We react in horror at past stories where the state inflicted prefrontal lobotomies on mental patients or forced intrauterine devices into economically poor women. To justify the bodily intrusion of forced vaccines, a great compensating good must be achieved at minimal cost to citizens who resist.

What would constitute that good? First, the vaccine would need to be highly effective, such that one dosage conferred a high degree of immunity for at least one to two years. Second, the vaccine would need to be safe, having been tested on every ethnic group, gender, and age, and been found to have no harm. But what if, like the vaccine for dengue fever, the vaccine made some people worse off? If that were true, mandatory vaccination would be hard to justify.

For many reasons, vaccine mandates will likely never work well in the United States. The present polarization of US politics hampers any national consensus about vaccination, and for vaccine mandates to work, the danger of the germ must be such a "clear and present danger" that even the dullest person could understand it, something like the ravages of Ebola.

The history of such mandates in America during Covid is enlightening. In 2021, New York City mayor Bill de Blasio required proof of vaccination for people to enter bars, restaurants, or sports arenas. De Blasio also required the vaccination of city workers who interacted with the public, such as police officers, bus drivers, and subway clerks. More controversially, he ordered that children over the age of five had to be vaccinated to enter public facilities.[2]

In retrospect, the moral justification of such vaccine mandates was shaky. After vaccines became widely available, the rationale for mandating them was even shakier. After half of Americans had experienced some form of the SARS2 infection, probably by the spring of 2022, all justification vanished.

One rationale for mandates in the workplace was the protection of fellow workers. But America famously learned in 2021 that vaccinated people could still be infectious and pass on the virus to other people.

Another rationale for vaccine mandates was to speed up herd immunity. But if variants of SARS2 could spread even among the vaccinated, why were mandates needed?

Covid hit African Americans especially hard, and as such, they were prime candidates for a good vaccine, but many African Americans did not believe the federal government usually had their best interests in mind.[3] Forcing them to take vaccines against their will? How would that encourage their trust?

As said, an argument for the mandatory vaccination of adults generalizes from the justifications for vaccinating all children.[4] One such justification is utilitarian: the vaccination of every child helps to protect not only the child, but all other children in the community. Another is the benefit to the child, say, of the DPT vaccine: parents are not permitted to forgo a great benefit to a child if it is easy to get that benefit without risk. Third, mandatory vaccination creates herd immunity, protecting vulnerable children with compromised immune systems who cannot get vaccinated.

Such justifications for the mandatory vaccinations of children are rational and altruistic, but not every parent is rational and altruistic. Moreover, what is true for children is not necessarily true for adults.

Mandatory vaccination in adults might create resistance effects, such as active rebellion against local ordinances and actively fostering measures to avoid vaccination. As such, policies of mandatory vaccination might paradoxically lead to lower rates of voluntary vaccination.

What about a college? Would it be permissible to require vaccination against Covid for all students before they arrive on campus? Many colleges already do so for mumps, rubella, and measles vaccinations. One poll by the Pew Research Center found that one-third of college students declined a vaccination for Covid.[5] Paralleling national fears in the same groups, only 22 percent of Black respondents and 37 percent of Hispanics said they would voluntarily take a Covid vaccine.

If the fear of severe disease and death can't motivate rational people to take a shot, why should the government force them to do so for their own good? Many will probably be sorry if they land in a hospital with Covid, but there should be limits to what government forces people to do for their own good.

But what about for the good of others? Well, the unvaccinated will get infected and more than 90 percent will survive, so eventually herd immunity will develop, regardless of how many get vaccinated.

Anti-vaxxer groups, such as Children's Health Defense, founded by Robert F. Kennedy Jr., and Texans for Vaccine Choice, fired early salvos against mandated Covid vaccines.[6] So popular did anti-vaccination sentiment become that in 2024, 10 percent of Americans considered Robert F. Kennedy Jr. to be a serious candidate for president. At the very least in America, mandatory vaccination would meet with great resistance.

NOTES

1. Michael Lederman, Maxwell Mehlman, and Stuart Youngner, "Require Vaccines for All to Defeat COVID," *USA Today*, August 10, 2020, 7A.

2. Joe Nocera and Bethany McLean, *The Big Fail: What the Pandemic Revealed about Who America Protects and Who It Leaves Behind*, Penguin, 2023, 237.

3. Jared S. Hopkins, "COVID Vaccine Trials Have a Problem: Minority Groups Don't Trust Them," *Wall Street Journal*, August 5, 2020.

4. Anthony Skelton and Lisa Forsberg, "Mandating Vaccination," in *The Ethics of Pandemics*, Broadview Press, 2020, 131–34.

5. C. Thigpen and Cary Funk, "Most Americans Expect a COVID Vaccine within a Year," Pew Research, February 2021.

6. Kerry Murakami, "Should Students Be Required to Be Vaccinated," *Inside Higher Ed*, July 10, 2020.

CHAPTER 15

Changes Accelerated by Covid

Some changes in America had already started before Covid, such as working occasionally from home, watching movies at home on streaming channels, and homeschooling kids. But Covid poured fuel on those changes, accelerating many and making some permanent. Some working parents (especially mothers) who wanted a better work-life balance found the changes preferable and they didn't want to return to working in offices after the pandemic subsided.

Anyone who travels to New York City, Portland, Seattle, San Francisco, or Atlanta today can see other big changes. America's epidemics of addiction and homelessness flooded the big cities of the United States with shambling, desperate people, often with three concurrent problems: mental illness, addiction, and homelessness. Attempting to treat such vulnerable people for Covid proved nearly impossible, and some of those who survived now suffer from Long Covid.

MEDICAL PROFESSIONALS QUIT

Even before Covid, many who worked in the health-care field felt burned out. Physicians in primary care often had to do paperwork for which they weren't paid, or were paid little, while specialists earned three times more. When for-profit hospital chains tried to speed up encounters to generate more revenue, some doctors quit, and for those who didn't, Covid came along and pushed many out early.

During the Covid pandemic, the ones who delivered the most care at the bedside—nurses and orderlies—were commonly asked to do too much, especially as for-profit chains took over hospitals and reduced staff to the barest levels, paying everyone as little as possible to maximize return to shareholders.

When Covid hit, such workers were expected to be heroes. Doctors in infectious diseases, pulmonary medicine, and cardiac (ECMO) support were put on the spot and often worked twenty-four-hour shifts, sleeping in nearby hotels rather than returning home and risk infecting their families.

PPE protocols were not yet fully developed. Prior to Covid, wearing an N95 mask required being appropriately sized for the mask. Once Covid began, taking time for proper sizing was discarded. People were given masks one day, told they didn't need them the next, then told a week later they needed positive pressure, whole-body suits. Worse, people without clinical backgrounds made such decisions. The whiplash effect on the frontline staff caused attrition among nurses and elderly physicians.

In general, about half of American physicians experience some level of burnout in their careers.[1] However, the Covid pandemic pushed some of these doctors over the edge, making them quit or even commit suicide.

In New York City, during the hard-hit wave in March 2020, two physicians who cared for Covid patients committed suicide.[2] One was Lorna Breen, who, after so many other doctors in New York City got sick, at one point was supervising two separate ER units. After getting Covid herself, Breen had a breakdown and returned to her native Virginia, where friends and family tried to take care of her. But caring for Covid patients had broken her, and at the end of April 2020, she killed herself.[3]

One explanation for the suicides of physicians during the pandemic was *moral distress*, a term in ethics that refers to the harm inflicted on one's integrity when circumstances force one to act unethically. In nursing, moral distress occurs when a nurse knows the right action to take, but orders prevent the nurse from doing so.[4]

In the spring of 2020 in New York City, twenty thousand patients died. During this time, Nathan Link, an ER physician, said, "Our staff had never seen so much death. Normally, a patient dying would be such a big deal, but when you start having a dozen patients die in a day, you must get numb to that, or you can't really cope."[5] Dr. Link characterized this numbness as "psychological distancing."

Aides in Kentucky public nursing homes, who made twenty-three dollars an hour, struggled with a lack of PPE and with demanding elderly patients and their families.[6] In such circumstances, where infection with Covid was ever-present, it's hard to think of oneself as a hero.

A related form of moral distress occurs with moral displacement, where a person's ethical code seems out of sync with those around him or her. It can occur when a medical worker is acting morally, even heroically, toward patients, and yet the patients are neither grateful nor cooperative, but actively hostile and seeming to despise the medical worker who is trying to help. One pulmonary doctor told me of repeatedly needing to treat Covid patients in the ICU who screamed, "I don't have Covid! I can't have Covid. It's a fake disease!"

WORKING FROM HOME

In March 2020, because of Covid, nearly half of the 143 million working Americans needed to try to work remotely from home for at least some of the workweek. Four years later, 80 percent of workers went back to working in person, but 10 percent still worked fully remotely and another 10 percent worked a hybrid schedule.

During Covid, whether you could work at home fully or partly depended a lot on your educational status. Low-paid workers with minimal education suffered the highest rates of infection, and afterward, they were still stuck working in person, especially in nursing homes, grocery stores, construction sites, and retail stores.

This new world of work reflects how Covid exacerbated class and racial inequalities. White and Asian workers were more likely to work in jobs where they could work partly or fully from home.

Given that such work—done remotely, from home or even a coffee shop—can occur anywhere, many Americans moved from high-tax states, such as New Jersey, California, and New York, to low-tax states, such as Florida, South Carolina, New Hampshire, and Alabama, or to recreation-filled states such as Colorado.

As mentioned, one group that benefited from the normalization of remote work was that of educated parents with children or those who cared for elderly parents. Although they were expected to offer the most resistance to returning to in-person work, Americans under the age of twenty-five came back easily and in greater percentages than middle-aged workers, perhaps because they lacked childcare responsibilities or because they missed the social life of offices.

Another group that benefited were people with disabilities, who no longer had to struggle with public transportation not suited to them or with out-of-date office spaces. This group benefited from fully remote work, which sometimes allowed them to do jobs not accessible to them pre-Covid.

Owners of coffee shops benefited from empty offices downtown. Many new coffee shops opened in suburbs and exurbs, allowing people to get away from their residences for a few hours to work undistracted. Because 60 percent of Americans drink coffee every day, new coffee shops started everywhere.[7]

No wonder in 2023 "Help Wanted" signs appeared everywhere for face-to-face jobs. Because of generous unemployment benefits, direct payments for childcare at home, and money saved from not commuting, many people continued to work at home and rejected face-to-face jobs.

DOING COLLEGE FROM HOME

Covid not only caused millions of kids in public schools to fall behind a year in reading and math, but it also damaged the work ethic of many professors and college students. Under the guise of nourishing a healthy "work-life" balance, the scales shifted from 75 percent work/25 percent life, to 50 percent work/50 percent life, or even 25 percent work/75 percent life.

Teachers and college professors discovered that being at home was like having continuous snow days while still getting paid. They were together with their spouses, kids, pets, and grandparents, and in too many cases, it beat working in offices. For teachers who lived on Staten Island and who taught in Queens, it saved them one-hour commutes each way.

Teachers and professors also discovered that no one was watching. It was one thing for supervisors to walk by classrooms and observe the teaching taking place there. It was another to stalk the teachers' online classes to see what they were doing and for how long. And the one thing that teachers or professors really hate is for any supervisor to take a deep dive into their teaching.

The truth is that 99 percent of the time (to which I can attest, having been an administrator myself), administrators rely on trust and professionalism, only dealing with problems that pop up and that can't be contained privately. As a result, many professors became accustomed to only teaching a few hours a day, to not commuting, and to having lots of time at home.

It wasn't just educators who liked working from home. Psychiatrists and radiologists set up home offices with secure, encrypted connections, enabling them to converse with patients or read scans on Zoom. Savants at Microsoft and Google realized that not only could they work from home, but that their home didn't need to be in expensive California; it could be in Idaho, Texas, or Tennessee, with less expensive costs of living.

Some students also learned to cheat while taking tests at home on Zoom. Because administrators feared mass exits of students, they encouraged professors to "give kids a break" on their tests and papers. Usually when students claimed illness or hardship, most got a break, and some became accustomed to asking for special treatment. As previously lamented, in K–12 schools, the resulting chronic absenteeism remains out of control to this day.

During the Covid pandemic, every university pivoted to online teaching, forcing professors to learn how to teach that way. My own university invested millions of dollars for cameras in classrooms to digitally record the class lectures. Four years later, classes are still being recorded (to the anger of many faculty members, who fear controversial classes could be subpoenaed), and students have become accustomed to missing classes and later watching the video recordings. To help students with disabilities and those who become sickened with ordinary germs, my administrators kept the recordings going. But these recordings do, in fact, encourage students to miss classes.

Scheduled meetings on Zoom replaced professors' in-person office hours. Although they were still required to post official office hours for talking to students, no administrator checked whether faculty members actually kept them, because administrators themselves held all *their* meetings on Zoom and came to campus as infrequently as possible.

The faculty senate at my university switched to Zoom meetings four years ago and never returned to in-person meetings. The same happened for the committee meetings of faculty.

Administrators meet other administrators almost entirely on Zoom, modeling this behavior.

As a result, we have created ghost campuses. The retention of students became a problem, as more and more wondered what the point was of attending empty campuses. Even the first two years of medical school, which is almost entirely comprised of classroom instruction, has gone either online or is now digitally recorded, so that when I pass a classroom in the medical school, a professor might be lecturing to seven students while the other 193 watch from afar.

Accelerating across-the-board absenteeism from K–12 schools, universities, and offices, people increasingly live their lives on social media. College students, even on campus, walk with heads down, staring at their cell phones or texting messages with their fingers. Everyone seems to be on social media around the clock.

Gone are the days when everyone attended a movie in person every other week. They all now watch streaming shows on Netflix, Amazon, Hulu, Disney, Max, Paramount, Peacock, ESPN, and so on. Departments try to attract students to courses with Instagram or Facebook postings.

Once upon a time, I could walk into my building at 9 a.m. on a weekday, look down a long hallway of professors' offices, and see that half had their doors open with a professor actually inside typing up a paper or talking to a student. Now it's a ghost hall, not just in my building but in almost every non-lab building on campus. When I on the rare occasion run into another professor, we stop and chat, so unusual is it to have in-person contact.

I experienced the same changes. I researched and wrote my last two books largely away from my office at UAB. People helped me in faraway places, reading drafts and chapters sent by email. Because of a special program I run for seventy college students pre-admitted to medical school, I see students socially more than most professors, but even with them, we've all cut back our face-to-face meetings. Students often resist coming to see me in my office and ask to meet on Zoom.

Covid also accelerated other changes, which medical sociologists will discuss one day, but curious readers can use this endnote for a list of eight more changes that Covid has probably made permanent.[8]

POST-COVID, UNHAPPY DEMOCRACIES

The United Nations regularly ranks the world's happiest countries. Critics might challenge the metric it uses, but it is surprisingly simple and effective: it asks citizens, on a ten-step ladder—where the lowest step represents the worst-possible life and the highest step the best-possible—how they see their lives.[9] Citizens of Nordic countries (Sweden, Denmark, Norway, Iceland, and Finland) consistently rank their lives high on that ladder, but in 2023, Americans ranked their lives fifteenth, and in 2024, their happiness fell to twenty-fourth.

What makes life in the Nordic countries so good? Trust in government, generous welfare benefits, rough economic equality, high literacy, wide-ranging personal freedom, and good public education, to name a few. Of course, most citizens in these countries also share a cultural history and political perspective, which counts for a lot.

Something clearly ails Americans. As the *U.N. World Happiness Report* notes, "In many but not all regions, the young are happier than the old. But in North America happiness has fallen so sharply for the young that they are now less happy than the old."[10] Perceived unequal life prospects, an increasingly hot planet, racial tensions, fears of immigrants, political brinkmanship, funding of weapons in foreign wars, unattainable homeownership, and the aftereffects of Covid have left many Americans feeling that bad things have happened in the past decade from which they will never recover.

Economic unease prevails everywhere. Four years after Covid began, many in Western democracies still feel that things aren't right. In 2024, Japan comes in fifty-fifth in happiness. One Japanese professor confessed to me in 2024 that, "Our youth aren't getting married or having children because they see such a bleak future for the next generations." Of course, fertility decreases with education, but something still seems amiss. Japan has the longest-living citizens in the world, but not enough young people are paying taxes to fund care for them.

In Australia and North America, many feel economic hardship: renters fear they may never be able to buy a home, the traditional sign of middle-class, economic security.[11] "Happiness also fell significantly in the country group [that includes] . . . Australia and New Zealand, by twice as much for the young as for the old." Of course, Great Britain and France experienced similar problems, and citizens there expressed dissatisfaction in their 2024 elections. Historically, such feelings have led to political upheaval.

NOTES

1. L. Dyrbye and T. Shanafelt, "A narrative review on burnout experienced by students and residents," *Med Educ.* 2016; 50: 132–49.

2. Noah Weiland, "Burnout among Health-Care Workers Soared after Pandemic Hit, CDC Finds," *New York Times*, October 24, 2023; Brittany Trang, "New CDC Campaign to Reduce Burnout in Health Care Workers," *STAT*, October 31, 2023.

3. Wring, 46.

4. American Association of Critical Care Nurses, "Moral Distress in Nursing: What You Need to Know," https://www.aacn.org/clinical-resources/moral-distress.

5. Lawrence Wright, "The Plague Years," *New Yorker*, 41–42.

6. Noah Weiland, "Burnout among Health-Care Workers Soared after Pandemic Hit, CDC Finds," *New York Times*, October 24, 2023; Brittany Trang, "New CDC Campaign to Reduce Burnout in Health Care Workers," *STAT*, October 31, 2023.

7. "Coffee Shop Industry Trends and Statistics in 2024," TOAST, https://pos.toasttab.com/blog/on-the-line/coffee-shop-industry-trends-and-statistics (accessed May 17, 2024).

8. (1) Touchless payments, either by tapping a credit card, by Venmo or Apple Pay, etc., in grocery stores, department stores, gas stations, or restaurants. (2) Online life—Facebook, FaceTime, Instagram, podcasts, YouTube, TikTok. Seniors who had never used Facebook or Instagram, who had never listened to a podcast or a recorded book, learned to do so to connect to their grandchildren. (3) Mental health problems, especially of young people. People tended to only post on social media the best aspects of their lives, which distorted what others think is a normal life, making them depressed that they, too, can't spend their spring break skiing in Zermatt. (4) Seeing people wearing face masks and thinking it's normal. (5) Fake online personal ads, aka "catfishing" and financial scams. (6) Delivery to residences of food, groceries, building supplies, and almost everything else, including pet food. (7) Fast food–like delivery of marijuana in cities such as New York and cities of the American West Coast. (8) Childcare becoming exorbitantly priced and/or hard to secure. Poorly paid workers decided the risk of COVID was too great, and post-COVID, they found higher-paying jobs. Subsidies to parents and childcare facilities ended, creating a crisis of a lack of available childcare.

9. United Nations, *World Happiness Report 2024*, https://happiness-report.s3.amazonaws.com/2024/WHR+24.pdf.

10. Ibid., 5.

11. Natasha Frost, "In Wealthy, Stable Australia, the Economic Gloom Is Proving Hard to Shake," *New York Times*, March 29, 2024, A23.

The Challenge of Long Covid and Disability

If you don't have it, you don't think much about it. If you do have it, you don't think about much else. Long Covid, defined by the CDC as "post-Covid conditions," lasts at least four weeks after illness and usually lasts much longer. In 2021, Congress recognized it under the Americans with Disabilities Act (ADA).[1] Those with Long Covid often call themselves "Long Haulers."

When science journalist Ed Yong interviewed a dozen health-care workers with Long Covid, he was shocked at how these workers had their symptoms dismissed by fellow workers.[2] Yong learned that significant numbers of doctors dismiss Long Covid as a fabrication. Canadian psychiatrist Jeremy Devine actually thinks vocal activist groups fabricated the phenomenon to get benefits, a view echoed by Johns Hopkins medical professor Marty Makary.[3]

Skeptics urge Long Haulers to "exercise out of it," when, in fact, exercise usually worsens Long Covid, creating post-exertional malaise. This common mis-advice led physiotherapists with Long Covid to found LongCovidPhysio, which cautions that Long Haulers should carefully allocate their energy each day.

FACTORS PREDICTING LONG COVID

After four years, scientists have come to better understand who gets Long Covid. People who had the most severe cases of Covid are most at risk for Long Covid, in part because severe Covid varies with age and comorbidities. If you contracted Covid at the age of eighty and you have both chronic obstructive pulmonary disease (COPD) and diabetes, you were not only more likely to die from Covid, but you were also more likely to later develop Long Covid.

Being overweight made you more likely to get sick with a Covid infection, as did being a smoker or having asthma, coronary artery disease, or COPD.[4] Women are 1.5 more likely to experience Long Covid than men, and white women more than women of color. Being unvaccinated dramatically increases the risk of Long Covid, in part because infection is likely more serious without vaccination.

Long Covid also occurs more often among Covid-infected people who did not take Paxlovid or monoclonal antibodies. You can get infected with Covid multiple times, and the more you do, the greater your risk of developing Long Covid.

PREVALENCE OF LONG COVID

The movement called Survivors Corps is a self-help and advocacy group for Long Haulers, with 187,000 members, most of them female. In England, a subgroup of Survivors Corps on Facebook for health-care workers with Long Covid has 1,400 members.[5]

One study in 2022 estimated that one in seven adult Americans who had Covid had to later stop working full-time or substantially reduce their working hours.[6] Some studies suggest that as many as one in thirteen American Covid patients became Long Haulers. Although this figure may seem high, if anything like it is true, then America has a budding public health emergency and a mass casualty event for its disability system.

Some cases of Long Haulers are heartbreaking.[7] At the age of twenty-eight, Nicole Bruno became a full-time caregiver to her thirty-year-old husband, a resident in neurology at the University of California at Irvine. She says that Covid "ruined his life. He cannot talk or walk and has 24/7 sensory deprivation."[8] Information designer Giorgia Lupi got Covid in Brooklyn in March 2020, and her journal chronicles her twenty-one different symptoms of Long Covid over the next 1,380 days.[9]

New York Times journalists followed radiologists as they examined the CT scans of several Long Haulers who had serious symptoms two years after their initial infection and discovered permanent scarring of the walls of the alveoli in their lungs.[10] None of these patients will return to their lives as they were before Covid.

The exact number of Americans suffering from Long Covid is hard to know. Before discussing estimates of Long Covid in America, let's discuss several factors that may have caused such large numbers of Americans to suffer from it.

First, America had one of the highest per capita rates of Covid in the developing world. Second, America had many unvaccinated citizens. Third, because of cultural battles, large numbers of people who tested positive believed that it was "brave" or "manly" to avoid medical treatment and just endure their symptoms.

Given the widespread belief among some that the dangers of Covid had been exaggerated to help President Joe Biden's campaign, it is understandable that people who originally believed this are also later reluctant to admit they have Long Covid. Indeed, it is possible that the self-recognition of Long Covid may be mediated by gender and race: in one clinic in New York City that saw 1,200 Long Covid patients, 80 percent were white, and 70 percent were female.[11]

In May 2022, a survey by the CDC's Covid-19 Emergency Response Team estimated that one in five Americans under the age of sixty-five who were diagnosed with Covid suffered from at least one medical condition that could be Long Covid. Among Americans over the age of sixty-five, the figure was one in four.[12] This figure only included Americans over the age of eighteen who had a diagnosis of Covid in records in some medical facility.

A review in the *Journal of the American Medical Association* of 120 studies of Long Covid in 130 publications found a high risk of bias, depending on how original cases of Covid were counted and how *Long Covid* was defined.[13] An early study by Chinese doctors found that 55 percent of Chinese infected with Covid in 2020 in Wuhan had Long Covid two years later.[14] These figures turned out to be way too high.

Given past patterns of blaming victims, it is especially likely that Long Haulers will be seen as malingerers, as hypochondriacs, and as lazy. When they apply for disability, they will likely get little sympathy.[15]

In March 2024, a new survey by the CDC found that only eighteen million Americans lived with Long Covid, or 6.9 percent of adult Americans; of these, nearly four million had Long Covid so bad as to be considered debilitating.[16] Even these numbers pose significant challenges to America's disability system.

It is not commonly recognized that among the 1,100,000 deaths in America reported as "death from Covid," about 3,500 were from Long Covid.[17]

Worldwide, both Covid infections and Long Covid cases are probably more common than realized. In developing countries, the burden of Covid is likely much worse than commonly reported, and so the numbers there of victims of Long Covid is also probably underreported.[18]

SYMPTOMS OF LONG COVID

The symptoms of Long Covid vary greatly and may last years. Too many Long Haulers experience symptoms lasting more than two years. The most common symptom is fatigue. Fatigue can be constant or episodic, occurring after even mild exertion. Vigorous exercise will leave some lying in their beds. Long Haulers describe excruciating decisions, such as whether to shower or have a long conversation with a colleague, whether to do laundry or walk the dog, but never both.[19] People who formerly danced professionally or who ran marathons became unable even to exercise.

With respect to fatigue, Long Covid seems to resemble chronic fatigue syndrome, now defined as myalgic encephalomyelitis or ME/CFS.[20] At one time, doctors thought that people suffering from ME/CFS were faking it, but no longer. Long Covid also resembles postural orthostatic tachycardia syndrome (POTS), a kind of dysautonomia characterized by palpitations, orthostatic intolerance, tachycardia, and fatigue.[21]

A seven-year study of seventeen ME/CFS patients compared them with twenty-one healthy subjects and found their exhaustion was physiological, not psychological.[22] Whether it's because the virus lingers in the body, or because it disrupts the mitochondria (the "energizers of the cell"), the body may be trying too hard to eliminate the virus, leaving ME/CFS patients exhausted.

The researcher discovered that the twenty-one ME/CFS patients differed from healthy patients because they had a "chronic activation of the immune system, as if the immune system was engaged in a long war against a foreign microbe, a war it could not completely win and therefore had to continue fighting."[23] Those suffering from Long Covid may have immune systems that are fighting similar, unwinnable battles.

The unpredictability of Long Covid challenges physicians. Symptoms can fluctuate in intensity and can come and go, making it impossible to predict how Long Haulers will feel the next week or the next day. This unpredictability can be frustrating and can destroy people's happiness, making it difficult to work, to maintain friendships, or even to complete mundane activities such as buying groceries, walking the dog, or doing the laundry.

The NIH has launched several studies of Long Covid. One remarkable finding is a loss of cognitive ability in people with sustained Long Covid. Infection with the original variant, hospitalization for Covid, admission to the ICU, a lack of vaccination, and the duration of serious symptoms all predicted serious cognitive deficits.

Subjectively, Long Haulers have complained of poor memory and "brain fog," which compared to the "pump head" feeling of patients after coronary bypass surgery and prolonged exposure to anesthesia. The first cognitive tests of 113,100 people with Long Covid in England discovered that, compared to people who never had Covid, Long Haulers lost six IQ points.[24] Those with ICU admission lost nine points of their IQ.[25]

Besides fatigue and cognitive declines, the third-most-common symptom of Long Covid is long-lasting respiratory problems. As a virus infecting people through the air, Covid severely damaged the lungs.[26] Such patients may have spent months on ECMO or on a ventilator and may never again be able to breathe without supplemental oxygen.

Dyspnea, or difficulty breathing, can be diagnosed in five grades, from the mildest, difficulty only with vigorous exercise, to the most severe, difficulty when dressing or leaving the house. For a small percentage of Long Haulers, dyspnea prevents them from working and should make them eligible for disability benefits (more on this below).

Finally, after the initial loss of smell and taste from Covid infection, some people with Long Covid never regain their sense of taste or smell or live with altered taste and smell. Damage to neurons from inflammation in the olfactory system explains this symptom, with some such patients having 75 percent fewer olfactory sensory neurons than healthy patients.[27]

Whatever the symptoms of Long Covid, the root cause is probably a continuing presence of coronavirus in the body.[28] Gerald Wong, a UCLA molecular genetics immunologist, believes that even fragments of the virus can make the immune system think it's still there and continue to war against it, creating a cytokine storm that can be more damaging than the Covid infection itself.[29]

Disability Benefits and Long Covid

In January 2022, America's Social Security Disability Insurance (SSDI) program paid out benefits to over nine million Americans. Most Americans know little about how SSDI works or its philosophical assumptions, but a looming crisis could change that.

SSDI is not the same as Supplemental Security Income (SSI), a program that helps the poor, or Workman's Compensation, which pays out for on-the-job injuries of workers who cannot sue.

SSDI has two distinct requirements for eligibility: financial and medical. Financially, SSDI is funded by people who work through deductions from their wages and salaries. This is important because SSDI, like Supplemental Security Income, has thresholds for minimal contributions: a minimum contribution over forty quarters, but unlike SSI, twenty of those quarters must have occurred in the ten years before applicants apply. (A "quarter" is a continuous three-month period of employment.)

Like SSI, benefits track contributions: the more one paid in, the more one gets back: in 2022, one could get as little as $100 a month or as much as $3,345 a month.

So, why will millions of Long Haulers fail to get SSDI? First, when they apply, they must prove they were not able to work for the previous twenty-two months. That means they can't have received unemployment benefits, because receiving such benefits implies that they would have worked if they could have.

Second, the issue for the administrative law judges who determine benefits is not whether applicants can do their *former* work, but whether they can do *any* work at all. (Maybe you can't teach philosophy anymore, but you can monitor security screens at an airport.)

Third, and here enters the medical requirement, judges who rule on SSDI need objective medical evidence: a positive Covid test, medical treatment for Covid, hospitalization for Covid, or best of all, getting treated in a special clinic for Long Covid. Overall, no medical test can prove or disprove Long Covid. Because symptoms are not easily testable, it's hard to prove to medical examiners.

Some people infected with Covid thought they had the flu or a cold and never got tested for Covid. When they later need to document having suffered from Covid, they will lack proof. It is the same for people who had Covid and decided to "tough it out," never seeking help from clinics or getting antiviral medicines. All of them, when they seek disability certification, will lack medical documentation.

At-home tests will not qualify as such evidence, even if people could prove when they took the tests and kept the results. When they fell sick with Covid, about thirty million Americans lacked medical insurance and often did not seek expensive medical treatment. Only a tiny number of patients have access to Long Covid clinics, which often having waiting lists a year long.

Bottom line: without proof of having Covid or being treated for it, Long Haulers will be unlikely to get SSDI benefits.[30] Consider the four Long Haulers below, who—since the virus infected them a year before—have not worked at all:

- Sharon, age twenty-six, after earning her MBA at the age of twenty-four, managed a Target for two years.
- Emma, age forty-five, was a nurse for ten years from age twenty-five to thirty-five, after which she became a home-maker, but she got divorced in 2021, returned to work, and then got sick with Covid.

- Jackson, age forty-nine, part-time piano tuner, short-order cook, waiter, bartender, and Uber driver, rarely reported income or paid Social Security taxes.

- Simona, age forty-three, became sick in April 2020 as a nursing home aide and stayed home after that. Although she never tested herself for Covid, ever since she got sick, she has had fatigue and muscle weakness. She never had medical insurance, and she has never seen a doctor about her condition.

None of these will likely get SSDI benefits: Sharon lacks forty quarters, Emma lacks twenty recent quarters, Jackson only reported income for twenty-five quarters, and Simona lacks any evidence to support her claim.

Of course, the above problems affect many other kinds of workers, including those in and out of work because of chronic medical problems. Changing the eligibility requirements for SSDI would have an enormous impact, but given America's increasing long-term debt, this change seems unlikely to occur.

One question in bioethics concerns whether SSDI benefits should be reduced for the unvaccinated. Although some disability judges may go outside the guidelines and hold smokers, drinkers, and addicted people responsible for their resulting disabilities (and thus deny or reduce their benefits), most judges do not.

It's so variable how Covid affects different people, and how much they could've done or not done to prevent infection, that it will be difficult to appraise how much any Long Hauler was responsible for getting infected. Moreover, we don't deny treatment for COPD or lung cancer to smokers, or deny liver transplants to alcoholics, or treatment for AIDS to people who had unprotected sex or shared needles, so we would be inconsistent to deny SSDI benefits to Long Haulers based on a lack of vaccination.

One social question may become political: How severe should the onus of proof be on Long Haulers to prove they cannot work?

What if they got infected before they earned good money? Will they only get the most minimal benefit?

We hope that the symptoms of Long Haulers will eventually mitigate, such that they can resume normal activities and work. But what if they don't? Even if four million of the eighteen million American Long Haulers never become normal again, that's a huge drain on the SSDI system. Can America afford to be compassionate to so many? If not, how will they live?

Essential workers during Covid had to work in person more often than professional workers, and as a result, they were more likely to get infected and thus more likely to develop Long Covid. Doesn't society owe them special consideration for disability benefits? What about health-care workers who became infected on the job, who later developed Long Covid, and who then could not work? Again, shouldn't a just society give them some benefits?

Will we repeat the mistakes we made with ME/CFS victims, blaming them for their symptoms? When the sister-in-law of journalist Ed Yong developed Long Covid, he started interviewing Long Haulers who had been told by doctors that their problems were "all in their heads." Female Long Haulers especially heard this explanation. As he started publishing about Long Haulers, he received dozens, then hundreds, then thousands of emails from Americans experiencing similar dismissals and abandonment by medical professionals.[31]

CONCLUSIONS

Long Haulers need several things. First, because America did a poor job preventing this virus from infecting so many, isn't this the time to acknowledge our failure and help those whose lives the virus continues to destroy? Moreover, given the reduction in worker benefits over the last decade, and given the creation of millions of gig workers, isn't it time to create a new disability system, one that's not just insurance for long-term, regular workers, but one that also covers workers suffering from unexpected disability?

Although it is not a topic popular with most citizens, perhaps Long Haulers will motivate politicians to take another look at America's disability system. It certainly does not seem adequate to handle the number of workers who become disabled in the normal course of things, and if Long Covid truly becomes a mass casualty incident for medicine, the disability system needs a real overhaul.

Second, Long Haulers desperately need more research conducted about their condition. When Congress held hearings about the need for funding, some Long Haulers used their GoFundMe or savings accounts to pay their way to Washington, DC, to testify. In February 2021, Congress allocated $1.5 million to study the causes of and treatment for Long Covid. Two years later, critics lament that the money largely gathered data on how many people suffer from Long Covid, their symptoms, and possible co-causes, but it did not fund any clinical trials of new drugs. For example, ClinicalTrials.gov lists 386 clinical trials for Long Covid, but only twelve now recruit participants to test drug interventions. Long Covid needs more new champions, such as Dr. Ziyad Al-Aly of Washington University School of Medicine in St. Louis, who has published twenty studies about Long Covid, motivated by online complaints of patients.[32]

After one promising study at Stanford was prematurely halted, the chief editor of *Lancet* lamented that this disappointment "adds to the dismal state of clinical research relative to the substantial burden of the condition."[33] She believes that one in ten people suffer from Long Covid after infection, and she continues to be amazed at the lack of research on the issue. Why is this so? She writes:

The reasons of course are manifold, including diagnostic uncertainty, lack of validated biomarker (which ideally would be easy to integrate into current clinical practice), multisystem conditions not easily falling into the current system of medical specialties, misogyny and other prejudices against groups particularly affected by long Covid, historical neglect of other postviral conditions such as myalgic encephalomyelitis/chronic fatigue syndrome, a societal and political wish to go "back to normal," limited interest of the pharma industry in repurposing low profit drugs, minimisation of long Covid because of insurance and disability costs and so on. Last but not least, the mistaken belief that long Covid is a psychogenic condition also hinders progress.[34]

Notes

1. Centers for Disease Control and Prevention, "Long COVID or Post-COVID Conditions."

2. Ed Yong, "Even Health-Care Workers with Long COVID Are Being Dismissed," *Atlantic*, November 24, 2021.

3. Jeremy Devine, "The Dubious Origins of Long COVID," *Wall Street Journal*, March 23, 2021, A15; Marty Makary, "The Exaggeration of Long COVID," *Wall Street Journal*, December 13, 2022, A17.

4. Pam Belluck, "Analysis Reveals the Biggest Risk Factors for Long COVID," *New York Times*, March 24, 2023, A20.

5. Ed Yong, "Even Health-Care Workers with Long COVID Are Being Dismissed."

6. Jenny Gross, "The Difficulties of Returning to Work with Long COVID Symptoms," *New York Times*, May 16, 2022, B4.

7. Ed Yong, "What Reporting on Long COVID Taught Me," *New York Times*, December 22, 2023, A16.

8. Nicole Bruno, "Long COVID, a 'Vicious Affliction,'" *New York Times*, January 28, 2024, A23.

9. Giorgia Lupi, "1380 Days with Long COVID," *New York Times*, December 24, 2023, 9.

10. Jeremy White et al., "An Inside Look at COVID's Lasting Damage to the Lungs," *New York Times*, August 28, 2023, A1, A12.

11. Daniela Lamas, "Why Are So Many of Our Long COVID Patients White Women?" *New York Times*, September 29, 2022, A22.

12. Pam Belluck, "Study Says One-Fifth of Infected Americans May Suffer Long COVID," *New York Times*, May 26, 2022.

13. Mirembe Woodrow et al., "Systematic Review of the Prevalence of Long COVID, Open Forum: Infectious Diseases," 10:7, July 2023, Oxford Academic.

14. Jia Tang et al., "Recent Advancements on Long COVID in China: A Narrative Review," *Int J Gen Med*, 16: 2585–93, June 19, 2023.

15. Allysia Finley.

16. Melody Schreiber, "'Alarming' Rise in Americans with Long COVID Symptoms," *Guardian*, March 15, 2024, https://www.theguardian.com/world/2024/mar/15/long-covid-symptoms-cdc.

17. Pam Belluck, "Long COVID Has Contributed to More than 3500 Deaths in the U.S., a Study Finds," *New York Times*, December 14, 2022.

18. David Wallace-Wells, "Which Countries 'Won' COVID," *New York Times*, April 6, 2024, A16.

19. Samathi Reddy, "Strategies for Long COVID," *Wall Street Journal*, May 16, 2022.

20. Mayo Clinic, "Myalgic encephalomyelitis/chronic fatigue syndrome (ME/CFS)," https://mayoclinic.org/diseases-conditions/chronic-fatigue/symptoms-causes/sys-20360490.

21. "Svetlana Blitshteyn: On the Front Line with Long COVID and POTS," *GroundTruths with Eric Topol*, May 20, 2024.

22. Pam Belluck, "Chronic Fatigue Study May Help with Long COVID," *New York Times*, February 24, 2024.

23. Dani Blum, "In COVID, Fatigue Remains a Confounding Symptom," *New York Times*, October 1, 2023, D19.

24. A. Hampshire et al., "Cognition and Memory after COVID-19 in a Large Community Sample," *New England Journal of Medicine*, February 29, 2024, 390:9, 806–17.

25. Al-Aly Ziyad and C. Rosen, "Long COVID and Impaired Cognition: More Evidence and More Work to Do," *New England Journal of Medicine*, February 29, 2024, vol. 390, no. 9: 858–60.

26. Jeremy White et al., "An Inside Look at COVID's Lasting Damage to the Lungs," *New York Times*, August 28, 2023, A1, A12.

27. Joseph Finlay, "Persistent post–COVID-19 smell loss is associated with immune cell infiltration and altered gene expression in olfactory epithelium," *Science Translational Medicine*, December 21, 2022.

28. Zoe Swank et al., "Persistent Circulating Severe Acute Respiratory Syndrome Coronavirus 2 Spike Is Associated with Post-Acute Coronavirus Disease 2019 Sequelae," *Clinical Infectious Disease*, 76:3, February 1, 2023 (published September 2, 2022); Sumathi Reddy, "A Key to Long COVID

Is Virus Lingering in the Body, Scientists Say," *Wall Street Journal*, September 8, 2022.

29. Nicole Karlis, "'Zombie' COVID-19 Fragments Linger for Some, Causing Severe Disease Outcomes, New Research Reveals," *Salon*, February 2, 2024.

30. For this discussion of disability benefits, I am indebted to Rhonda Curry of Louisville, Kentucky, a lawyer who has specialized in helping clients get SSDI benefits for many years, and who also worked for decades helping administrative SSDI judges adjudicate cases.

31. Ed Yong, op. cit.

32. *TIME* magazine, "100 Most Influential Doctors and Scientists," vol. 203, nos. 15–16, 2024.

33. Ursula Hofer, "Where Are the Long COVID Trials?" and "Medicine: Rapid Expert Consultation on Crisis Standards of Care for the COVID-19 Pandemic," *Lancet* (editorial), August 2023, https://www.thelancet.com/journals/laninf/article/PIIS1473-3099(23)00440-1/fulltext.

34. Ibid.

The Mysteries of Good and Bad Covid Leadership

Late one night in February 2020, in a recorded phone call, American president Donald Trump told famous journalist Bob Woodward that SARS2 spread more easily than the seasonal flu.[1] At this time, Trump emphasized to Bob Woodward that, "It's more deadly than even your seasonal flus," and then repeated to Woodward, "This is deadly stuff."[2]

Failures of leadership exist when the leader adopts the wrong philosophical framework or has people around him telling lies. Another kind of failure occurs when a leader is paralyzed during a crisis and can't make any decisions.

But what happened with Donald Trump during Covid may have been worse, because to say that he "failed to lead" is too simple. In retrospect, two important facts cry out for explanation. First, Trump was famously a germaphobe. At formal events where he was required to shake many hands in a line, an aide followed him with hand sanitizer.[3] This was a man who feared germs and who did not want to get sick.

Second, this was a man who did not want to leave the presidency. His attempt to block the official transfer of power in January 2021, after he lost the election in November 2020, is well-known. During his campaign for the Republican nomination for president in 2023 and 2024, he vowed to increase the powers of the president to go after his enemies. Since leaving the White House, he has done everything in his power to return to the presidency.

That is exactly what philosophers such as Michel Foucault feared would happen during a pandemic; Foucault taught that the state always tries to control and normalize citizens through the use of police, education, and medicine.[4] Italian philosopher Giorgio Agamben, after Covid deaths mounted around Milan in February 2020, witnessed Italy's prime minister Conte lock down the entire country for months, despite protests from libertarians and businessmen.[5] Foucault and Agamben both feared that power corrupts politicians, who then want to extend that power indefinitely.

Many critics of Trump accuse him of far more than having the wrong priorities or of being a poor leader. Far more seriously, they accuse him of constantly following his own pursuit of lifelong power while ignoring the real job of the president.

Thus, it's a great mystery why Trump did not seize on this great opportunity during Covid to become "President for Life." What could have been easier? The mystery deepens when we realize that critics constantly lambasted Trump for doing too little, too late, as when he shut down planes from China only after thousands of Chinese had already flown into America, and he only shut down flights from Italy and Europe after other thousands—many carrying SARS2—had entered the country. Why did he not assume greater powers when he could have taken them?

We know that Trump knew for certain that the virus was highly contagious and dangerous, yet he publicly stated the opposite. On February 24, he told the nation that, "The coronavirus is very much under control in the USA. The stock market is starting to look very good to me."[6]

GOOD LEADERS

It's illuminating to contrast how Trump led with how other leaders in the world led during the Covid pandemic. Governor David Ige and his lieutenant governor effectively led the state of Hawaii to contain the virus and mitigate the economic harms of the lockdown there. He told visitors to stay away, and its Tourism Authority paid for visitors to fly home. He even shut down travel between its seven inhabited islands.

Women also led well: Consider Jacinda Ardern in New Zealand, Angela Merkel in Germany, and Nicola Sturgeon in Scotland.

On March 25, 2020, Jacinda Ardern instituted a monthlong, "level 4" lockdown: everyone had to stay at home, schools and businesses closed, and only hospitals, groceries, gas stations, and pharmacies could remain open. People could only interact inside their families and exercise locally. They could only go to pharmacies or grocery stores while wearing masks and by staying six feet apart.

Ardern adopted the goal of Zero Covid: "Our elimination strategy is a sustained approach to keep it out, find it, and stamp it out."[7] Her texts were blunt: "This message is for all of New Zealand. We are depending on you. . . . Where you stay tonight is where you must stay from now on . . . it is likely level 4 measures will stay in place for a number of weeks."[8]

Because of how she led during the Covid pandemic, as well as how she responded to the terrorist killings of Muslims at Christchurch by a white supremacist, liberals around the world have called her "Saint Jacinda," seeing her as an anti-Trump, feminist, compassionate, effective leader, a woman so progressive that she gave birth while in office and took a child with her to address the United Nations.[9]

By June 8, 2020, and by her being transparent and eager to work with scientists, almost all New Zealanders followed her to Zero Covid. In August 2020, Trump, irritated by comparisons of him to her, criticized Ardern, saying New Zealand had had a "big jump" in cases, when, in fact, it had nine new cases. Trump said this when the United States had tens of thousands of new cases every day and had 170,000 deaths from Covid, while Ardern's New Zealand had only twelve deaths.[10]

However, as Covid dragged on, Ardern should have pivoted on Zero Covid to Focused Protection. New Zealand's economy depended on tourism, and it needed the tourists to come back.

When Ardern tried to impose vaccines on the country by making its policies harsh on anti-vaxxers, her "we're all in this together" mantra broke down into a two-class system, causing resentment among those who saw forced vaccination as a violation of their civil liberties, a "jackboot of authoritarianism."[11] A three-week sit-in in the spring of 2022 by protestors at New Zealand's Parliament, resembling truckers' protests in Canada, sank her popularity. In January 2023, she abruptly resigned, looking haggard and saying she had "nothing left in the tank."

In Germany during the Covid pandemic, Prime Minister Angela Merkel quickly established three principles: (1) all two hundred public and private German labs would produce the test for SARS2, (2) the test would be free for all Germans, and (3) all other testing would be sidelined for the rapid turnaround of SARS2 tests.[12]

After testing, results in Germany came back within twenty-four to forty-eight hours. If negative, Germans could do as they pleased. If positive, they had to self-isolate. With its quick results, Germany did not have as many problems as America with flattening the curve because it's easier to get citizens to isolate for one to two days than for two weeks.

Like many other European countries, Germany restricted travel, mandated social distancing, required masking, and closed nonessential businesses. Merkel matter-of-factly explained the virus and its consequences, resulting in widespread support, so

German hospitals were not overwhelmed like American hospitals were.

In Scotland, Nicola Sturgeon led similarly; she ramped up testing, restricted social gatherings, and got the National Health Service prepared to treat Covid patients, especially those in nursing homes. As one journalist summed up her efforts:

> *Throughout the Covid pandemic, Scotland's then first minister, Nicola Sturgeon, posed as a cross between Mother Teresa and John Knox, compassionately but sternly protecting her people, as much from Boris Johnson's mayhem as from the virus.*
>
> *As a result, Scottish lockdowns were longer and harsher than those in England. People in Scotland were constrained to within five miles of their homes when no such restrictions existed south of the border. Mask requirements persisted far longer, and vaccine passports were demanded more widely in Scotland—not just for large events, but even for "sexual-entertainment venues," which are not known for facilitating mass gatherings.*[13]

RON DESANTIS

Although he may lack the charisma of other well-known politicians, Ron DeSantis is no doubt an intelligent person, one known as a policy wonk. Of all the world's leaders, he studied Focused Protection and even invited authors of the Great Barrington Project to Florida to discuss their ideas with him.

DeSantis ultimately decided these authors were correct and employed Focused Protection in Florida, to great effect. He protected nursing homes, closed schools as infrequently as possible, and kept businesses as open as possible. As mentioned, during the Covid years, two million Americans thought life was better in Florida than elsewhere. Undoubtedly other factors drove this movement, such as lower taxes, Miami being a center of Spanish-speaking culture, a supportive medical structure for retired Floridians, and the availability of full employment.

As of June 1, 2024, New York State's roughly twenty million people had roughly 6,400,000 confirmed cases of Covid and roughly fifty-three thousand Covid deaths. Florida's roughly twenty-three million people had roughly 7,500,000 confirmed cases and roughly eighty-six thousand Covid deaths.

Of course, Florida's median age tops New York's by three years, but also 1.5 million people over the age of sixty-five and a half million over the age of seventy-five moved to Florida during the Covid pandemic. Thus, given who's most likely to die of Covid, even with the best policies, more Covid deaths would have occurred in Florida.[14]

What is remarkable is that with comparable Covid statistics, Florida's schools and businesses stayed open, its cities prospered whereas New York's floundered, and despite hurricanes and global warming, millions still moved there. Ron DeSantis must be given credit for much of that.

ANTHONY FAUCI

Anthony Fauci did his best in an impossible situation. For four previous decades, he had led the National Institute for Allergies and Infectious Diseases. Starting during the early years of HIV/AIDS, the gay community at first hated him, but later, he became their partner in accelerating the development of antiretroviral drugs.

His tenure in science earned him the respect of his peers, but his position was perilous under Donald Trump, who had inherited him from previous administrations. Fauci seemed always torn between saying what the best science indicated, in all its complexity, and what the president wanted him to say.

Fauci recognized that for Trump, more was at stake than preventing infections and deaths from Covid. Most notably, he knew that Trump wanted to project himself as a strong leader and didn't want to damage the economy. Therefore, Fauci must have been constantly torn between the Prime Directive and Trump's desire to look strong in a flourishing economy.

Unfortunately, Fauci came to symbolize for the far right all that they hated about Covid restrictions. In February 2020, even though it looked bad in Wuhan and Milan, he erred badly in saying the threat of SARS2 in America would be "miniscule."[15]

Truth to tell, SARS2 also could have faded in the spring, like the swine flu of 1976 in America, or like SARS1. As for SARS1, for mostly unknown reasons, nine months after it first appeared, it disappeared as a threat to public health. So SARS2 in 2020 might have run the same course, disappearing after the hot summer months.

In February 2020, Fauci also said the wrong thing about wearing masks ("There is no reason to be walking around with a mask"). In saying this, had he caved to Trump's antipathy to masks? He later walked back his statement about masks, saying he had made that claim then because he feared there wouldn't be enough masks available for medical workers. But this then irritated everyone who interpreted it as misleading Americans to protect medical workers. Some asked: Will he lie again to protect medical workers?

As previously discussed, Fauci thought of SARS2 too much like the flu and not enough as a different kind of virus, was too slow to detect asymptomatic spread, and seemed surprised that vaccinated people could both spread SARS2 and get reinfected.[16]

When Trump famously suggested, in a nationally televised press conference, injecting bleach or horse dewormer to rid SARS2 from infected people, Fauci looked chagrined, but he would not publicly contradict this boss. Fauci probably knew that if he did, he would be sidelined. Perhaps by staying in office, he hoped to temper some of Trump's wilder impulses as well as help the nation get through Covid.

Fauci was thrust into an impossible position, serving under a president obsessed with the stock market and with bad news about Covid, but also serving professionals demanding exactitude under uncertain conditions.

Fauci made mistakes, as would anyone in the same position (and as Rochelle Walensky later learned during her brief tenure as head of the CDC). Some of his mistakes were philosophical, in not appreciating the harms to children of extended lockdowns and the benefits of Focused Protection.

It may be helpful to his critics to try to imagine themselves in his place at the start of 2020, when China had taken the extraordinary step of quarantining eleven million citizens, and later, when the BBC showed army convoys in northern Italy taking body after body of elderly Italians to graveyards. What message would they have given the American public then?

It is also helpful to contrast Fauci's tenure with that of CDC director Robert Redfield. The latter was distrusted by virtually everyone, even those inside the CDC, and he will go down in medical history with Dr. Wilmer Krusen, director of Philadelphia's Department of Health during the Great Flu of 1918, who allowed the Liberty Loans Parade to be held in Philadelphia.

IMAGE VERSUS REALITY IN LEADERSHIP

Pandemics create rare opportunities for politicians to lead. Like being attacked in war, the nation yearns for a strong leader with definitive answers. One lesson about leadership during pandemics is that it's easiest to lead if you have one and only one goal, and in the case of SARS2 and Covid, that one goal was preventing infections. Ardern achieved amazing results, as did Nicola Sturgeon, but both also risked turning the state into a libertarian hell. Still, people in New Zealand, Scotland, and Germany largely trusted their female leaders, and as a result, these women achieved good results.

Some American politicians rose to the occasion better than others. In New York, Andrew Cuomo, in the spring of 2020, seemed to be the national leader whom everyone yearned to follow. He held daily briefings on the virus and mitigation efforts, and he spoke with authority, seemingly following the science and the advice of experts in public health. As a result, and throughout the summer of 2020, his approval rate among New Yorkers was 77 percent.[17]

Again, it was easier to lead and lead forcefully if the only goal was containment of the virus through lockdowns. But Cuomo badly misjudged one aspect of the pandemic, making a horrendous mistake that he later tried to cover up, and that was sending patients from nursing homes who entered hospitals sick back to their nursing homes, in some cases still infectious. As a result, these returning patients became an amplification system for the virus in their original nursing homes.

Cuomo later tried to disguise the number of deaths from Covid among nursing home residents by not counting their deaths if they died in hospitals. But no other state counted Covid deaths that way. Thus, where New York State officially reported only sixty-five thousand such deaths, the true number was nearly twice that.[18]

Of course, Cuomo had other liabilities. He ignored the public health advice around him and later had to resign because of charges against him of sexually harassing women.

California governor Gavin Newsom did not fare much better. Both Cuomo and Newsom had presidential ambitions, and they used the pandemic to gain national attention as leaders, but Newsom's fell apart when an alert waiter photographed him eating indoors at the elite French Laundry restaurant with a group of eleven other people, none of them wearing masks, and all violating the governor's own mandates for social gatherings and mask-wearing. He also kept California schools closed far longer than any other state, resulting in horrific setbacks in learning, especially in poorer districts, and continuing problems of absenteeism.

Britain's Boris Johnson suffered from hypocrisy like Newsom's, which began with a Christmas party in December 2020 at the prime minister's residence, where lots of alcohol was consumed and staff did not socially distance. This occurred when Johnson had closed most pubs in Great Britain.

There is a saying that the cover-up is often worse than the crime, and Johnson got in trouble with Parliament for lying about the event. London Police handed out 126 fines about eight gatherings involving Johnson where the Covid rules had been broken. Like Trump, whom his leadership resembled in some ways, Johnson didn't seem to take the virus seriously and tried to project an image of himself as a heroic leader.

In June 2023, on the eve of a report from a committee in Parliament recommending removing his privileges, Johnson resigned, calling the report a "witch hunt" against him.[19]

And alas, Nicola Sturgeon was later also brought down by a financial scandal involving her husband and their personal use of 600,000 pounds of the Scottish National Party (SNP). At first, she abruptly resigned, but then later she was arrested. Although these financial improprieties had nothing to do with her leadership during the Covid pandemic, it does show that few politicians are perfect.

Like Ardern, Angela Merkel quit as chancellor of Germany in 2021, perhaps because managing the Covid crisis, along with the immigration crisis in the European Union, and all the other problems of Germany over sixteen years, took a toll on her and her family.

One of the great undocumented costs of Covid, and the stresses of managing it, was burnout among health professionals and politicians who took their jobs seriously, whereas Trump and Johnson, who in many ways did not, did not burn out and never wanted to leave office.

DELVING INTO TRUMP'S INNER MIND

As said, those around Donald Trump knew that he hated germs, and that they frightened him. Former chief of staff Mark Meadows writes:

> *Trump is a massive germaphobe. [In meetings with him] if a person coughs . . . that person is made to leave the room immediately. [Trump] famously kicked Mick Mulvaney out in full view of the press for letting out an uncovered cough. Every time he went on a trip, even in the days before anyone had heard of Covid-19, he would go through buckets of hand sanitizer.*[20]

We know from Matthew Pottinger and Anthony Fauci that Trump knew that SARS2 was more dangerous than the flu and that it was highly infectious. So, why did Trump act as if SARS2 and the Covid infection it caused was nothing more than the common cold?

Despite his fear of germs and of SARS2, Trump hated to wear masks in public or in the White House. Why? The obvious answer is that he thought it made him look weak. He ridiculed Joe Biden for wearing a mask in public during his 2020 campaign for president. He encouraged people around him not to wear masks at public events, resulting in the infamous amplification system in the Rose Garden.

This reveals a desire to appear strong and manly. Being infected with SARS2, becoming sick with the Covid virus, must have shaken Trump to his core because it made him look both weak and foolish, two things he never wanted to be seen as. He also knew that his base wanted to see him as a strongman, an invulnerable leader who would protect them, so Trump played to that image.

Behind all of Trump's approaches to Covid was that he wanted it to "be no big thing." He had hope, in early February

2020, that it would go away in the spring or summer months, just as previous viruses had faded, including the swine flu of 1976.

Of course, he didn't want Covid to affect the stock market or the American economy. There is a saying in bioethics: "always follow the money" to understand an issue, and although money doesn't explain everything, we should never ignore how physicians get paid and how that influences their behavior. Similarly, how responses to Covid affected the American economy mattered a lot to Trump.

It is also no mystery why Trump didn't embrace the Focused Protection strategy of Ron DeSantis. DeSantis kept Florida's economy running and convinced Florida's voters—many of them Trump supporters—that a certain number of Covid deaths—for example, sixty to seventy a day—was acceptable to keep everything open, from schools to Disney World.

But in 2020, Trump saw DeSantis as his likely rival for the Republican nomination for president, so he couldn't give his *bête noire* any credit, much less embrace the plan of a policy wonk dubbed by Trump as "De Sanctimonious." Yes, Trump wanted to keep the entire America economy humming the way Florida's hummed, but he wanted all the credit for doing so, and he certainly didn't want to share any credit with DeSantis when both men officially resided in Florida.

The idea that Trump cared more about not looking weak than getting sick from Covid is borne out by the sensational events that took place during the last months of the presidential campaign in 2020 between Trump and Biden. Starting in September, Trump wanted to downplay the seriousness of the virus, probably aware of how much his administration had botched its response to it.

Things began to go downhill after the celebration in the Rose Garden of the White House on September 26 of the nomination of Amy Coney Barrett for the US Supreme Court, where dozens of people became infected, including Barrett's former boss, the president of the University of Notre Dame. Almost all those present curried favor with Trump and did not wear a mask or socially distance.

According to Mark Meadows, hours after that celebration, Trump tested positive for SARS2, a fact kept secret in his presidential campaign.[21] Meadows writes that Trump looked tired, with eyes red around the edges—an unusual look for Trump. Trump himself demurred, saying he hadn't slept well and might be coming down with a cold.

Three days later, on September 29, Trump debated Joe Biden on national television, so it is obvious why he kept his Covid infection secret—he did not want to look weak. Meadows affirms that he did not want to be seen as canceling the debate because he was ill. A second Binax test came back negative, but as Meadows watched Trump around the White House, he saw the president had dark circles under his eyes and moved very slowly, as if struggling to act normal. At that point, Meadows writes, "I decided that I should act from now on as if he was positive."[22] Deep down, Meadows knew the truth.

By debating Biden, as many have argued, Trump endangered Biden and the entire staff staging the debate, a pattern he would repeat with his Secret Service protection detail. Among those prepping him for the debate were Chris Christie, Hope Hicks, and Jared Kushner, all of whom soon became infected.

The next day, on October 1st, Trump attended a fundraiser in New Jersey, unmasked, with donors. By then, as many as forty-eight others who'd had contact with Trump were infected: First Lady Melania Trump; Kellyanne Conway; Mark Meadows; Matt Gaetz; physician Ben Carson; and a few US senators, campaign staffers, and Republican fundraisers.

When Trump returned from the fundraiser, Meadows writes, "He was pale, exhausted, and nearly asleep on his feet."[23] Even Trump began to admit that he wasn't feeling well and that he felt weak. Sean Conley, a doctor of osteopathic medicine and a naval commander, was Trump's official White House doctor, and he quickly gave Trump a PCR test, the kind most people got, where a long swab goes up the nose. An hour later, they knew for certain that Trump was positive for Covid.

Mark Meadows immediately scrambled to get emergency approval for treatments for Covid that had not yet received FDA approval, especially REGEN-COV, a powerful form of monoclonal antibodies. Meadows did not want to tell the top brass at the FDA who it was who needed emergency "compassionate use." The FDA resisted until finally Meadows broke down and told them the president needed REGEN-COV.

On October 2nd, on what was probably the seventh day of his Covid infection, Trump gave in and announced to the public that he had tested positive for the virus. At this point, the original plan was to treat him in the White House. This is important because it's a baseline for determining just how sick Trump was and how much his later "Superman" image was a lie.

Meadows writes that about 11 p.m. that evening, he and Dr. Sean Conley rigged up a four-poster bed so they could start an IV drip to administer the REGEN-COV. By the next morning, Trump's oxygen levels had dropped to 86 and seemed to be still going down, so Dr. Conley began to give him oxygen.[24] More worrisome to Conley was that tests had shown that, despite being infected with SARS2, and unlike most people with Covid, Trump still had no natural antibodies fighting the coronavirus, which meant, Conley feared, that without the monoclonal antibodies, Trump might fare very badly.

Conley soon realized that in trying to treat one of the most powerful and obstinate men in the world, in his bedroom with unproven treatments and with the nearest emergency room miles away, he was out of his depth as an ordinary osteopathic physician who was neither a pulmonary nor an infectious disease specialist. Nevertheless, when Conley and Meadows suggested a transfer to Walter Reed Hospital, Trump resisted. Why? Meadows writes:

"From his first speeches [on Covid], he sought to project an air of strength. He wanted people to know that although this virus might be bad, it was nothing that the American people couldn't handle."[25] As Meadows looked at him, Trump still had red streaks in his eyes, and for once, the president was not at his desk, but sitting up in bed dressed in a T-shirt. Meadows feared the worst. About this time, Meadows later wrote, "The President's vitals were very concerning."

Trump kept resisting going to Walter Reed, fearing it would make him look weak. Son-in-law Jared Kushner later confirmed that Trump did not want to enter Walter Reed Hospital because he thought it would make him look weak.[26]

But Meadows brilliantly turned the "Don't look weak" argument against Trump, arguing that he would look a hundred times weaker being transferred prone on a gurney than walking to a helicopter under his own power. Feeling terrible and not wanting to be wheeled out on a gurney, Trump relented.

After he dressed for a very public walk to the helicopter, he carried a symbolic briefcase weighing about ten pounds and stuffed with inconsequential papers, but at the last moment, he was too weak to carry it and put it down.

Just how sick was he? We will never know, but it's revealing that President Trump became sick at the same time as Melania and Hope Hicks, but neither of them needed to go to a hospital. It seems like Conley and Meadows had reasons to urge Trump to go to Walter Reed.

Inside Walter Reed, Trump became paranoid that the doctors would describe him as being "very sick" or secretly take pictures of him, and so he asked all of them to sign nondisclosure agreements.

In the hospital, doctors aggressively treated Trump, giving him both REGEN-COV and remdesivir, an antiviral drug that inhibits viral replication, and presumably, continuous oxygen through a nosepiece. He also received the steroid dexamethasone, given to reduce inflammation in the lungs.

During his hospitalization, Trump wanted to give the appearance of being unaffected by the coronavirus: he released pictures of himself working at a desk and signing papers (one of the papers in the photo was blank).

On October 4, he made doctors let him briefly leave Walter Reed in a SUV with Secret Service men inside, waving to crowds and television cameras before returning inside. For this, he was later criticized for exposing his Secret Service detail to infection, but it seems to have never occurred to him that he might be doing so or that he didn't have the right to so expose them.

After a deceptively upbeat press conference by Sean Conley, Mark Meadows huddled with reporters "off the record" and told them that, "The President's vitals over the last 24 hours were very concerning and that the next 48 hours will be critical in terms of his care." This might have been a rare slip of truth about the president's real condition, caused by an exhausted chief of staff at the limits of his abilities.

Trump immediately bawled Meadows out for puncturing his carefully constructed strongman facade. In his memoir, Meadows tries to walk back his statement, attributing it to sleep deprivation (even though he had just mentioned he had slept the night in a room down the hallway from Trump).[27] In any case, it is clear that as soon as he got back to Trump's room in the hospital, where Trump had been watching the live press conference on TV and immediately heard Meadows's remarks, Trump yelled at Meadows, accusing him of making a "rookie mistake."

Undoubtedly Trump's true intentions were revealed by the *New York Times* when it was reported that he'd made several phone calls claiming that he would leave the hospital and feign weakness, then suddenly rip off his shirt to reveal a Superman suit underneath.[28] In his memoir, Meadows tries to do damage control about this story, claiming it was just a joke.[29]

Although Trump did not actually do his "Superman" routine, it clearly appealed to his ego and his desired image, so upon his return to the White House, when he got to the balcony of the South Portico, he posed for pictures while taking off his mask and saluting the crowd. An hour later, he posed a video message that said:

We're going back to work. We're going to be out front. As your leader, I had to do that. I knew there's a danger to it, but I had to do it. I stood out front. I led. Nobody that's a leader would not do what I did. And I know there's a risk, there's a danger, but that's OK. And now I'm better and maybe I'm immune. I don't know. But don't let it dominate your lives.[30]

So, there you have it. As Trump tweeted several times, "Don't be afraid of Covid. Don't let it dominate your lives."[31]

Deconstructing Trump's messages to Americans, we get: "Real men don't fear little viruses. Men should tough it out and go on with their manly lives. Don't give in to being sick and weak." As Lawrence Wright writes in *The Plague Year*, "But the image of the maskless President spoke to people, especially his base. He appeared defiant, masculine, invulnerable."

Undoubtedly, these messages caused harm. As Lawrence Wright writes, "The President's bravado . . . caused many more fatalities," such as that of thirty-seven-year-old army vet Richard Rose, who refused to wear a mask, caught Covid, and died three days later.[32]

Surely for some people, being macho was lethal. Not everyone had medical insurance. Not everyone would get the triple combination of steroids, oxygen, remdesivir, and REGEN-COV that Trump received, which at the time was experimental and only given as "compassionate use"—and then only because Meadows had pushed FDA commissioner Stephen M. Hahn to the brink.

Donald McNeil Jr., in his book *The Wisdom of Plagues*, discusses what the "poor leadership" of Donald Trump cost America in excess deaths. Comparing the leadership of Justin Trudeau in Canada and Angela Merkel in Germany, McNeil concludes:

> *But by early 2023, as the pandemic wound down, we in the United States had suffered almost twice the per capita death rate of Germany, and almost three times that of Canada. In a population the size of ours—330 million—that means that we could have lost only 560,000 Americans instead of 1.1 million if we had handled ourselves well enough to land somewhere between German and Canada. What cost those 540,000 Americans their lives was poor leadership.*[33]

Think about how Trump's example in the fall of 2020 affected a seventy-four-year-old white man named John living on Social Security on a small pension in rural Albertville, Alabama. Suppose John had also waited six or seven days before thinking about entering a hospital for treatment. But in John's case, it wouldn't be Walter Reed, but his local community hospital, which would lack both pulmonary and infectious disease specialists. In other words, by taking the manly stance, John could have developed severe Covid and possibly have died, or John might only have mild lung damage but then Long Covid for years. For men like John, following Trump's example could have hurt them badly.

WAS ANYONE A GREAT LEADER DURING COVID?
Covid exposed the faults of many national leaders. Boris Johnson got caught partying with his friends without masks or social distancing, flouting the rules he imposed on his countrymen, then lying about what he had done. Andrew Cuomo sounded great on television, but he made terrible decisions about nursing homes, causing many deaths there, all before problems surfaced

as a result of his handsy approach to women. Jacinda Ardern led well in New Zealand, but she continued the lockdowns for far too long, then burned out over the pushback. Nicola Sturgeon in Scotland also led well, but a financial scandal with her husband got her in trouble. Jair Bolsonaro was such a clown in Brazil that afterward he fled the country for Florida, and when he was forced to return to Brazil, he was charged with abetting a *coup d'état* and abuse of presidential powers.

No leader was perfect, and none were truly great during Covid. Perhaps, as Socrates concludes at the end of the *Meno* about teaching virtue, whether someone arrives in adulthood with virtue, or acts as a great leader during a pandemic, is truly "a gift of the gods."

ANSWERING THE MASTER QUESTION

Covid leaves us with several mysteries: Did the coronavirus emerge from a well-intentioned project in a Wuhan lab? Did authorities suppress a well-known strategy of harm reduction for reducing the toll of fighting the virus on Americans? Did a germophobic president consistently downplay the lethal effects of the virus but not seize the opportunity to invoke martial law in a public health emergency, granting himself extraordinary powers?

I once had a mentor who was allergic to bees but who vowed that his life wouldn't be ruled by such an allergy. So, he kept bees in his backyard and sometimes donned a protective suit while tending the bees.

My guess is that Trump did fear the virus, especially when he got sick, but he was ferociously determined not to let it get the better of him. After he watched alcohol kill his older brother, he became a teetotaler, and just as he wouldn't let alcohol better him, he also resisted a virus doing so.

In his memoir, Trump's attorney general William Barr agrees with this assessment for two reasons. First, he asserts that Trump believed he would be easily reelected, so he saw no need to grab continuing power the way he later did in urging the mob to storm the Capitol on January 6, 2021. Second, Barr claims that Trump:

> *had a deep need to project himself as a strongman. In this instance, that meant adopting a defiant bravado to show he was not going to be pushed around by a mere virus.*[34]

Thus, to declare a Public Health Emergency over the coronavirus would have given it too much power, in the president's mind, both over Trump and over the country. He needed to dismiss its importance—its power over him and over America—and tell everyone to "man up" and ignore it. Maybe he was so determined to minimize it that it never occurred to him to go the other way and exaggerate its danger in order to become "President for Life."

And in this regard, America got lucky.

NOTES

1. Bob Woodward, *Rage*, Simon & Schuster, 2020, xix–xx.

2. Bob Woodward, *Rage*, xix–xx.

3. Mark Meadows, *The Chief's Chief*, All Seasons Press, 2021, 155.

4. Michel Foucault, *The Birth of the Clinic: Archaeology of Medical Perception*, originally, *Naissance de la Clinique—une archéologie du regard medical*, Paris: PUF, 1963.

5. Giorgio Agamben, *Where Are We Now?: The Epidemic as Politics*, October 8, 2021, Valeria Dani, trans.; Christopher Caldwell, "The Coronavirus Philosopher," *New York Times*, August 21, 2020.

6. Reuters, February 24, 2020, "Trump Says Coronavirus Under Control in the U.S."

7. C. Taylor, "How New Zealand's 'Eliminate' Strategy Brought New Coronavirus Cases Down to Zero," CNBC.com, May 5, 2020, https://www.cnbc.com/2020/05/05/how-new-zealand-brought-new-coronavirus-cases-down-to-zero.html (retrieved August 18, 2020).

8. C. Taylor, "How New Zealand's 'Eliminate' Strategy Brought New Coronavirus Cases Down to Zero," CNBC.com, May 5, 2020, https://www.cnbc.com/2020/05/05/how-new-zealand-brought-new-coronavirus-cases-down-to-zero.html (retrieved August 18, 2020).

9. Yan Zhuang, "The Highs and Lows of a Prime Minister Who Became a Global Star of the Left," *New York Times*, January 19, 2023.

10. Eleanor Ainge Roy, "Trump Calls Out New Zealand's 'Terrible' COVID Surge, on Day It Records 9 New Cases," *Guardian*, August 17, 2020.

11. Damien Cave, "How COVID's Divisions Tarnished a Liberal Icon," *New York Times*, January 19, 2023.

12. Melissa Eddy, "Traveling to Germany? A Free COVID Test Awaits," *New York Times*, August 6, 2020, A8.

13. "Scotland's COVID inquiry is destroying the case for lockdowns," https://collateralglobal.org/article/scotlands-covid-inquiry-is-destroying-the-case-for-lockdowns/.

14. Graham Brink, "How Old Are Floridians? Five Charts Tell the Story," *Tampa Bay Times*, January 11, 2024.

15. Anthony Fauci, "miniscule" risk.

16. Linsey Marr, "Yes, the Coronavirus Is in the Air," *New York Times*, August 3, 2020.

17. *The Big Fail*, 204.

18. *The Big Fail*, 209.

19. "UK's Boris Johnson and the 'partygate' scandal," Reuters, June 15, 2023, https://www.reuters.com/world/uk/uks-boris-johnson-partygate-scandal-2023-06-15/.

20. Mark Meadows, *The Chief's Chief*, All Seasons Press, 2021, 155.

21. Mark Meadows, *The Chief's Chief*, All Seasons Press, 2021, 151.

22. Mark Meadows, *The Chief's Chief*, All Seasons Press, 2021, 163.

23. Mark Meadows, *The Chief's Chief*, All Seasons Press, 2021, 170.

24. Mark Meadows, *The Chief's Chief*, All Seasons Press, 2021, 176.

25. Mark Meadows, *The Chief's Chief*, All Seasons Press, 2021, 176.

26. Jared Kushner, *Breaking History: A White House Memoir*, Broadside Books, 2022.

27. Mark Meadows, *The Chief's Chief*, All Seasons Press, 2021, 200.

28. Mark Meadows, *The Chief's Chief*, All Seasons Press, 2021, 211.

29. Mark Meadows, *The Chief's Chief*, All Seasons Press, 2021, 211.

30. Trump's quote upon leaving the hospital.

31. Tweet by Donald J. Trump.

32. Richard Rose's death, on following lead of Trump.

33. Donald McNeil Jr., *The Wisdom of Plagues: Lessons from 25 Years Covering Pandemics*, Simon & Schuster, 2024, 40.

34. William Barr, *One Damn Thing after Another: Memoirs of an Attorney General*, William Morrow, 2022, 454–55.

CHAPTER 18

Why Operation Warp Speed
Almost Didn't Happen

THE OFFICIAL STORY

The official view about Operation Warp Speed is that it was a predictable success of capitalism and American biotechnology, and that the next time a dangerous germ appears, America can just give Big Pharma billions of dollars again, and it will produce another great vaccine.

Pfizer and Moderna had research facilities, but Novavax, a small startup in Maryland, did not. And many of the key ingredients for making and distributing one hundred million dosages of new vaccines were made in China, which was not eager to let them leave.

Fortunately, Trump stayed out of this biological Manhattan Project, letting Moncef Slaoui, a retired head of vaccine development at GlaxoSmithKline, and General Gustav Perna, handle things.[1] Secretary of the treasury Steven Munchin pulled ten billion dollars from the CARES Act to fund research into new vaccines. In case its vaccine worked, he also gave the Jenner Institute one billion dollars for ten million doses of the AstraZeneca vaccine.

Operation Warp Speed, and vaccines created by the nonprofit Jenner Institute, did save lives, perhaps as many as 3.2 million Americans.[2] But there is more to this story than the public knows, especially the unlikely path to the success of the new vaccines.

THE REST OF THE STORY

In fact, it's a miracle that the mRNA vaccines were created in the first place. The two researchers who laid the groundwork for them, Katalin Karikó and Drew Weissman, who deservedly won the Nobel Prize in Medicine for creating them, were treated horribly by the University of Pennsylvania and by their peers there.

The history of medicine is littered with stories of brilliant researchers whose colleagues scorned their new ideas. Fellow physicians thought Ignaz Semmelweis crazy for suggesting that their dirty hands spread German measles among poor women whom they examined as they lined up in stirrups for gynecological inspections. Stanley Pruisner, who ultimately won the Nobel Prize in Medicine and Physiology, could not get fellow scientists to accept the idea that a protein could be infectious. (He believed that prions caused spongiform encephalopathies such as mad cow disease.) American ophthalmologists for decades dismissed laser surgery for eye problems as Russian quackery. Similarly, for decades everyone in medicine knew that stress and mental issues caused ulcers, not *Heliobacter pylori.*

Karikó and Weissman had the idea of basing vaccines on mRNA technology, an idea that was considered crazy and radical by both the University of Pennsylvania and other scientists who were trying to make vaccines, and who instead were using DNA to make them, not RNA. As one medical journalist summarized:

DNA has two strands of nucleotides that wind around each other like a twisted ladder, making it durable. . . . Inside the cell, mRNA only sticks around a short while before it is eliminated. And the body has developed elaborate methods to ward off the molecule. To Karikó, mRNA was the perfect molecule—it only needed to get inside the cell's walls to create proteins, not all the way into the nucleus, like DNA.[3]

The chair of neurosurgery at Lenox Hill Hospital, David Langer, a former student of, and collaborator with, Karikó, said that her research was always a long shot, one that took years to achieve good results, and that could easily have been fruitless. "It begs the question of how many others aren't being recognized for their work," Langer said. "Michael Jordan was drafted third, Tom Brady was drafted 199th, you can say 'how did people miss them,' too," Langer said. "The story is that she [Karikó] persevered."[4]

One of her key breakthroughs was to enclose the RNA in a lipid nanoparticle to protect the unstable molecule until it reached a desired location, whereupon the lipid dissolved. A similar idea has recently gained ground among other researchers of synthesizing and modifying water-soluble macromolecules (synthetic and natural) to deliver drugs to specific targets in the body.[5]

After Karikó won the Nobel Prize, the University of Pennsylvania made millions from its patents on her research and hypocritically celebrated her as if she were its cherished professor.[6] Yet Penn never supported her research, and before she won the Nobel Prize, the university had demoted her and cut her pay.[7] Amazingly, she was also never tenured at Penn, only working there as an adjunct. After winning the Nobel Prize, she quickly left Penn to accept an offer of a full professorship at Szeged University in her native Hungary.

Science journalists Joe Nocera and Bethany McLean nicely sum up her contribution: "Even with Moderna's and Pfizer's efforts, even with Operation Warp Speed, if it hadn't been for Karikó's dedication, it would have taken much, much longer to develop a Covid-19 vaccine. Meaning that tens, if not hundreds, of thousands more people would have died."[8]

The world owes a lot to her, and not much to the University of Pennsylvania. The RNA technology behind the Covid vaccines should lead to further medical breakthroughs. It's also true that the world got lucky that Karikó persevered under such horrible conditions, which few other researchers would have done.

NOTES

1. Joe Nocera and Bethany McLean, *The Big Fail*, 280–85.

2. Paul Offit, "For the Next Pandemic," *National Geographic*, February 2024, 17.

3. Gregory Zuckerman, "After Shunning Scientist, University of Pennsylvania Celebrates Her Nobel Prize," *Wall Street Journal*, October 4, 2023, A1.

4. Gregory Zuckerman, "After Shunning Scientist, University of Pennsylvania Celebrates Her Nobel Prize," *Wall Street Journal*, October 4, 2023, A1.

5. See the research of UAB researcher Eugenia Kharlampieva at: https://www.ekharlamgroup.com/.

6. News Release, "Katalin Karikó and Drew Weissman, Penn's Historic mRNA Vaccine Research Team, Win 2023 Nobel Prize in Medicine," *Penn Medicine News*, October 2, 2023, https://www.pennmedicine.org/news/news-releases/2023/october/katalin-kariko-and-drew-weissman-win-2023-nobel-prize-in-medicine.

7. Megan Zahneis, "Penn Demoted Her: Then She Won the Nobel Prize," *Chronicle of Higher Education*, October 5, 2023.

8. Joe Nocera and Bethany McLean, *The Big Fail*, 306.

CHAPTER 19

Future Problems and Positives

POSITIVE #1: AMERICA'S SOARING ECONOMY

As described previously, the $1.9 trillion American Rescue Plan Act in 2021 followed the CARES ACT of 2020. These two acts and several smaller ones injected $4.52 trillion into America's economy, forestalling a recession. It was also one of the greatest investments in infrastructure in American history since World War II. Unappreciated by critics, it became an unexpected silver lining of the Covid pandemic.

Even though America avoided a recession, and even though its economy now fares better than those of most developed countries, most Americans in 2024 view their economy negatively. This may illustrate Bobby Duffy's *The Perils of Perception: Why We're Wrong About Nearly Everything*, which documents how many people misperceive important aspects of life, such as how often other people have sex or how many children are born without their parents being married.[1]

Because many upper-middle-class Americans didn't do much during Covid, they saved money. Such people now do makeup travel to class reunions, taking their grandchildren to Disney World and booking destination/adventure travel on cruise ships or with Road Scholar. Such rebound spending partly explains the resurgence of America's economy (and it helps Europe's economy, as well).

PROBLEM #1: AMERICA'S INFLATION AND SOARING DEBT

The infusion of trillions of dollars of new money into America's economy caused inflation, which continued after the pandemic ended and worries average Americans. Although pre-Covid, a movement had existed to make fifteen dollars an hour the minimum wage in most states, Covid made that movement moot, as so many people had left the workforce that twenty dollars an hour became the default average in many cities. With generous unemployment benefits (which sometimes exceeded the pre-Covid wages of some workers), people became accustomed to making more. Wages rose everywhere, but so, too, do did prices. Rents soared after pandemic restrictions were lifted.

Once upon a time, the American public cared about the national debt. Now it's not even on the list of its top five concerns. But Covid dragged America much further into debt: in 1992, America's debt was 46 percent of the Gross Domestic Product (GDP), but in 2024, it is 96 percent, nearly twice the average of other advanced countries. America's borrowing is so vast that, given the supremacy of the dollar in the world's currency, it could jeopardize the world's economic security. And its debt-to-GDP ratio will rise from today's 96 percent over the next thirty years to 166 percent.[2]

Worse, political polarization has several times in the last few years degenerated to brinkmanship and risking default. Should America miss the payments on its interest due, the world's financial system would wobble, and international stability would suffer.

POSITIVE #2: WE KNOW WHAT WORKS

First, masks work. Yes, they can be irritating to wear, but we must realize what we are taking risks when we shun them. First, they only work if we wear them in the right way. We need N95 masks that fit well, and we should never wear the mask with most of it pulled down and just covering our mouths, or worse, our chins. Why is that? The main goal of wearing a mask is to limit, not absolutely prevent, viral particles from entering our lungs and mucosa. No mask will be an absolute barrier against that entry of such particles. For that, we would need a plastic hood with a separate ventilation motor.

Second, we should ventilate, ventilate, ventilate if germs are being spread in the air. Although the importance of improved ventilation in fighting viruses has been suggested by people as different as Monica Gandhi, Ezekiel Emanuel, and sociologist Zeynep Tufekci, it hasn't filtered into any national consensus.[3] But it should. Besides stockpiling good PPE, better ventilation may be the easiest, most practical way to protect K–12 kids in schools and students in colleges from future bad germs.

Third, we should protect the most vulnerable first. At least 75 percent of frontline workers during the Covid pandemic were minorities. Pay special attention to nursing homes. Use Focused Protection. Beware false positives on tests, as well as putting healthy patients on units full of patients who really have the virus, thus causing new patients to be infected. (This happened with Binax tests, which had some false positives.)

Fourth, we should limit large events like the Liberty Loan Parade or Taylor Swift concerts, where thousands gather close together and can be amplification systems. "Studies showed that about 70 percent of patients infected with SARS-COV-2 wouldn't spread the virus any further, but about 5 percent of infected individuals without masks could account for as many as 80 percent of all subsequent cases, mostly the result of super-spreading events."[4]

Fifth, we should stockpile the reagents for PCR tests, PPE, and synthetic swabs that will be needed when the next pandemic hits. Don't rely on foreign manufacturers, who can hoard supplies for themselves. Don't depend on China or anyone else for chips for computers or essential chemicals for tests. True, since 2006, we had the Strategic National Stockpile of N95 respirators and surgical masks, but no one checked them for mold or age, so many of them proved useless. (Despite this obvious precaution, it appears that once again, we are not stockpiling enough.)[5]

PROBLEM #2: NEW VIRUSES

In April 2022, virologists detected a new, highly virulent flu virus, H5N1, in a farm in Newfoundland, Canada, and later discovered that it had infected wild birds, which spread the virus across Greenland and the United States.[6] To stop H5N1, American authorities in 2022 killed ninety thousand birds. Nevertheless, migrating birds in 2023 carried H5N1 down the west coast of South America, where it crossed over to sea lions, killing twenty-four thousand of them. By late 2023, it had rounded Cape Horn and traveled up the east coast of South America, through Argentina, through Uruguay, and to Brazil, killing thousands of elephant seals along the way.

What is important about this virus is that first, no previous virus had spread this way down the coasts of the Americas, nor had any infected marine mammals along such coasts. Like the early stages of SARS2, we still don't understand a lot about H5N1.

Then, in 2024, it was detected in American dairy cows. It had also already infected a man in Chile and then four workers on American dairy farms. Faced with criticism from scientists lamenting America's missteps over early testing for Covid, the USDA on April 24, 2024, began testing lactating cows moved across state lines, a small part of the total.

In April 2024, fragments of the virus were detected in the milk of American dairy cows on the shelves of American grocery stores. The agency testing did not say if the virus was active or dead, but it assured the public that the milk supply was safe. In May 2024, the virus was detected in beef tissue for the first time, but again, the Department of Agriculture said that eating beef was safe.

The US Department of Agriculture has always been beholden to the food industry, and it is not exactly a consumer watchdog. It has been slow to sound alarms about outbreaks of lethal O157:H7 *E. coli* in contaminated beef and organic produce, which causes seventy-eight thousand illnesses each year and at least forty deaths.[7]

With mutations caused by antigenic drift, crossover to humans was possible. But unwilling to cause a panic among American consumers, the US Department of Agriculture resisted testing all cows for H5N1, repeating the same mistakes of the past and leaving America in an epistemic black hole about how fast the virus was spreading and to whom. Preliminary genetic analyses of samples indicated that dairy cows in America could have been infected as early as January 2024 or even a month before.[8]

Farms are ideal for the crossovers of such viruses, with many kinds of animals crowded together, as well as farmworkers. So far, farms have been reluctant to have their cows tested, and because many use undocumented workers, such workers also fear cooperation with government testing that could potentially make them stop working.

Dangerous medical research could also be a source of new, crossover viruses. In May 2024, the White House started new rules to govern gain-of-function research on viruses and other dangerous microbes that might create another pandemic.[9] Many researchers applauded the new oversight and found it reasonable. It also seemed to be an indirect acknowledgment that SARS2 might have been the result of gain-of-function research in bat viruses that went awry.

Because no one can predict where a coronavirus will land in the body and stay, xenografts from pigs ("swine") have become more ethically problematic. We know that viruses jump mostly to humans from bats and pigs ("swine"). The possibility of a coronavirus jumping from pigs to humans, through the portal of an immune-protected, transplanted kidney inside a human patient who then leaves the hospital and interacts with people in his community, has now become real. An American left a hospital in Boston in 2024 with the kidney of a "swine" that may or may not carry viruses inside of the person's body. (It is impossible to sterilize a kidney in an autoclave and kill all viruses without also killing the kidney.)[10] A grandmother also left NYU Langone Hospital with a pig kidney, the fourth such patient to receive such a xenotransplant.[11]

Of course, it's impossible to guarantee that any transplanted pig kidney is completely free of viruses, and pigs are well-known sources of viruses that can mutate and harm humans. Whereas research on known dangerous germs is done in a P4 containment lab, people with transplanted pig kidneys walk out of hospitals, potentially carrying new viruses deep inside them, as if nothing could be dangerous about having the organ of a pig living inside their bodies.

Who knows what viruses may mutate and grow inside an immune-protected swine kidney deep inside that patient's body? And who knows if he, or other recipients of swine xenografts, will not be human portals of dangerous new viruses for humanity? Given the havoc created by SARS2, shouldn't there be more transparency and accountability for surgeons who perform xenografts?

Nevertheless, in terms of monitoring the danger of new viruses infecting humans, the safety of xenotransplantation is not on the radar screen of most IRBs. This is because the ethical issues of xenotransplants are almost entirely defined as opposition from People for the Ethical Treatment of Animals (PETA), whose views most meat-eating Americans don't care about. But Americans do care about preventing another pandemic.

POSITIVE #3: SOME DEMOCRATIC COUNTRIES KNOW HOW TO LEAD

Other developed, democratic countries modeled how to confront a pandemic successfully. Australia's Covid death rate was only one-tenth of the US rate.[12] Sweden kept almost everything open and had the same low death rate.

The democracies of the Pacific Rim also fared well during Covid, undoubtedly because they had so much prior experience with other pandemics. A panel of scientific experts led Japan's response to Covid, which fared exceptionally well until the Omicron variant hit. Even then, with 80 percent of its population vaccinated and despite having the world's oldest population, it had only seventy-three thousand Covid deaths among its 123 million citizens.

Similarly, South Korea responded exceptionally well to Covid, with quick drive-through testing sites and efficient contact tracing. With fifty-two million people, it had only thirty-six thousand Covid deaths. Similarly, Taiwan, with twenty-four million citizens, had only fifteen thousand Covid deaths.

And New Zealand kept Covid at bay, recording only about 2,500 deaths among its five million people, a remarkable achievement. And given the size of its population, at nearly twenty-seven million, Australia also did exceptionally well in allowing fewer than twenty thousand Covid deaths.

The above statistics show that the world doesn't need dictatorships to successfully fight pandemics. Although it's true that Singapore's authoritarian regime allowed only two thousand Covid deaths among its six million citizens, Singapore's population roughly compares to that of New Zealand, and both had about the same number of Covid deaths. But New Zealanders today are far freer than citizens of Singapore.

PROBLEM #3: POLITICIZATION OF MEDICINE AND SCIENCE

Although there is much to learn about what went wrong with American's response to Covid, whether future leaders can learn anything from our mistakes, and then correct them, is doubtful. Should another dangerous germ appear, Americans are so tired of Covid, and so polarized about the facts and policies concerning it, that I doubt whether any kind of consistent, evidence-based, unified response could occur.

Progressives read the *New York Times* and the *Washington Post*, and they watch MSNBC or CNN. Conservatives read the *Wall Street Journal* and watch Fox News. Progressives think lockdowns worked, that Focused Protection was fringe science, and that there is nothing to the Lab Leak Theory; they dismiss news about bad reactions to vaccines as aiding anti-vaxxer lunatics. Conservatives tend to dismiss Long Covid as hysterical hypochondria and think Covid was no big deal.

Almost 90 percent of Americans believe that Covid left us more divided than before. Everyone in America in 2024 seems to see themselves as having legitimate grievances. Certainly, the current fashion of identity politics plays a role, which tends to pit one group against another and make the other group respond angrily. Philosopher Kwame Anthony Appiah may espouse cosmopolitanism, but in America in 2024, he has few takers.[13]

If a new pandemic starts, as Donald McNeil urged, we should "go early, and go hard" to contain it, but does America presently have the political will to do so? I doubt it. First, if you are going to employ lockdowns, go all the way as early as you can. Yes, that could mean quarantining some people, although probably not as drastically as what China did. If the germ is dangerous, then half-hearted measures will be just as bad as no measures.

Countries such as Vietnam and New Zealand went hard early and kept their infections low. Australia, Taiwan, and Hong Kong employed quarantines with similar results. The Pacific Rim countries learned from their experience with SARS1 and other infections originating in China or India.

But now arises an ethical issue that will break American hearts and test the moral mettle of its leaders. For quarantines to be effective, no exceptions can be made. Consider what not only China, but the democratic country of Japan did: both blocked their citizens who were traveling abroad from returning home. For many such citizens, this meant years of involuntary absence from home.

America was more softhearted. In January 2020, fourteen thousand passengers arrived in America every day from China, most of them Americans. We evacuated the Americans from the cruise ship *Diamond Princess* and failed to adequately quarantine them in California, especially when Trump's minions met them at airports without wearing PPE and hence, spread infections to local California towns.

In April, the Trump administration announced that flights from Europe would soon be stopped, so massive numbers of Americans scrambled to fly home. But this was done without coordination with the CDC or government agencies, so the resulting lines and mobs at Atlanta's and New York's airports became amplification systems among the travelers, who then spread their infections across the continent.

Similarly, in the future, I don't see American politicians as being able to withstand the pressure of families who want their sons and daughters, or grandparents, returned to the United States during a pandemic.

POSITIVE #4: mRNA VACCINES

Like statins for cardiovascular health or semaglutide for weight loss, mRNA vaccines may turn out to be one of the great medical inventions of the century.

The new mRNA vaccines possess many advantages over traditional vaccines. As proven by comparisons with the AstraZeneca vaccine for Covid, vaccines that do not need to be grown in chicken eggs, or that do not rely on inactivated or dead virus, are safer than traditional vaccines. This means fewer adverse reactions, fewer cases of anaphylactic shock, and fewer deaths from vaccination.

Second, the new mRNA vaccines can be designed and manufactured at greater speed than traditional vaccines. Of long-term interest, they can also be produced more cheaply than traditional vaccines.

The real power of the new mRNA vaccines can be seen in Moderna's new research into the deadliest viral diseases suffered by humans around the globe, especially HIV, the Ebola family of viruses, dengue fever (an epidemic now in South America), malaria, and Zika.[14] The future of vaccines now looks very bright.

PROBLEM #4: BROKEN TRUST IN PUBLIC HEALTH

We need officials running the CDC, the FDA, and the NIH who can be trusted, and for this reason, such appointments should be like the head of the FBI, not varying by presidential administration. Of course, it would also help immeasurably to have a president who could lead during a pandemic by following the evidence and communicating honestly.

We have learned not to trust businesses that run cruise ships. A passenger had already died of Covid a week before on the *Diamond Princess* cruise ship when the *Ruby Princess* cruise ship left Sydney, Australia, on March 8, 2020, with 2,670 passengers and 1,146 crew members on board. The same cruise line operated the *Grand Princess of California*, which had a Covid death on March 4, 2020, such that it returned to Oakland for testing, where twenty-one people tested positive. The ship's 3,533 passengers and crew then endured quarantine until March 25, when many passengers went to Travis Air Force Base for testing and further quarantine.[15]

Eleven days after the *Ruby Princess* left Australia, six hundred people on board had contracted Covid, and twenty-eight then died. An Australian judge found Princess Cruise Lines liable for the deaths and allowed a class-action lawsuit against it, concluding that, "To proceed with the cruise carried a significant risk of coronavirus outbreak with possible disastrous consequences, yet they proceeded regardless."[16]

In Denmark, citizens trust their government and live happy lives. Over 80 percent got vaccinated and then got the booster. Trust has become the most precious asset any Western government can have.

POSITIVE #5: SOCIAL EPISTEMOLOGY

Up until recently, most citizens had no interest in epistemology, the branch of philosophy that deals with how we know statements to be true. And in truth, the field over the last century has become mired in arcane, internal squabbling over pet theories and minute points. But something recently changed, after Facebook, Instagram, Twitter (X), TikTok, and group emails emerged. Almost simultaneously, cable news split along severe political lines, with the multicountry Murdoch empire (Fox and Sky News, the *Wall Street Journal*, London's *Times*, HarperCollins, and 20th Century Fox Studios) pushing a far-right, conservative agenda, with MSNBC, CNN, and others pushing a liberal, leftist agenda.

Abstractly, we would all agree that knowing truth matters, that people who tell the truth are valuable, and that institutions that tell the truth can be trusted. In the ethical theory of virtues, a person who tells the truth has integrity and moral weight.

Despite these abstract claims, today truth is under siege from every quarter: in competing against each other for students, colleges are under pressure to present themselves in the best possible light, which means cranking up the PR machine and suppressing anything bad, such as rapes on campus. Cable news is under pressure to get the most viewers, so easy-to-understand, simplistic, sensationalist stories beat complex, hard-to-understand coverage.

Powerful new tools of artificial intelligence will blur truth going forward. The MIT Museum in Cambridge, Massachusetts, in 2023 already had a movie that looked completely accurate and real, showing the first human to walk on the moon dying there and President Nixon giving a sad speech about his death.

In talking to the public about germs during pandemics, truth has sometimes been a casualty for no malicious motive but other than that, "the whole truth and nothing but the truth" does not often lend itself to simple statements. Life is complex, fighting pandemic germs is hard, and such fights involve balancing many competing values.

When Covid first emerged, both Fox and CNN lacked the resources, or the sensitivity, or both, to really cover the beginnings. Only BBC, the British Broadcasting Company, reliably covered the daily events in Wuhan: the closing of the wet market, the quick building of the massive hospital complex, and the quarantine inside Wuhan province of eleven million Chinese. Even when the virus hit Milan and northern Italy, and army convoys were carting bodies to cemeteries, the BBC was the major and most accurate source of news about Covid.

Thus was born the new field of social epistemology. It is now more important to teach young people, and young citizens, how the truth can be found and who provides it. And that has become a very big challenge, because more and more young people do not watch any kind of news—Fox, CNN, or the BBC—at all, but they get everything they know about the world from social media.

PROBLEM #5: COVID MAY ALWAYS BE WITH US

Much as everyone wants Covid to disappear forever, the situation has morphed from pandemic to endemic. During the last twenty years, a neuroscience major has been the ticket for many premeds into medical school. For the next twenty years, that major will be immunology. And with that major will come the study of Covid and Long Covid.

The reason for this is that the coronavirus quickly creates variations, and in their evolutionary struggle to survive, some variants will surpass others, becoming more infectious or infecting more people. Although existing vaccines and natural immunity will protect most people from serious illness or death, new variants may evade such immunity, and new vaccinations will be necessary.

So, annual shots will be needed for Covid, just like for influenza. Moreover, just as the flu picks off the medically frail and vulnerable, so Covid will add another enemy for the medically vulnerable. Added to the sixty thousand Americans that flu kills every year, there may be another fifty to sixty thousand that Covid kills.[17] And if Covid and its variations are always with us, then Long Covid will be with us, too, creating new challenges for neurologists and experts in infectious diseases.

FINAL NOTE: REMEMBERING THE PANDEMIC

In 2034, how will Americans remember the Covid-19 pandemic? How will we remember how we responded to it? If nothing else, I hope the readers of this book take away the message that balancing different values in fighting pandemics is not just a medical decision, but a much more general one of public policy. Fighting disease and death is one value, but preventing business failures, overdose deaths, and years of loss of learning in kids are other values. The Prime Directive followed blindly caused too much harm. Choosing the right trade-offs among these values is not a medical decision, but a complex ethical one, one for which doctors and medical officials have no special wisdom.

Notes

1. Bobby Duffy, *The Perils of Perception*, Atlantic Books, 2018.
2. "Budgetary Blindness," *Economist*, May 4, 2024, 16–18.
3. Monica Gandhi, 133–34; The COVID Crisis Group, *Lessons from the COVID War*, 172–74; Zeynep Tufekci, "Why Did It Take So Long to Accept the Facts about COVID?" *New York Times*, May 7, 2021.
4. Gottlieb, 222.
5. Sean Michael Newhouse, "Is the strategic national stockpile ready for the next emergency? GAO says no," *Government Executive*, May 24, 2024.
6. Apoorva Mandavilli and Emily Anthes, "Concern Increases as Evolving Bird Flu Infects More Mammals," *New York Times*, April 25, 2024, A1–8.
7. Josefa Range, "Epidemiology of *Escherichia coli* O157:H7 Outbreaks, United States," CDC: Emerging Infectious Diseases, 1982–2002, vol. 11, no. 4, April 2005.
8. Apoorva Mandavilli, "U.S. Spread of Bird Flu Could Date to 2023," *New York Times*, April 25, 2024, A9.
9. Carl Zimmer and Ben Bueller, "White House Tightens Rules on Research That Could Risk Pandemic," *New York Times*, May 8, 2024, A20.
10. *New York Times*, April 4, 2024.
11. Karen Weintraub, "Heart pump, pig kidney, save grandmother," *USA Today*, April 16, 2024, A1.
12. Damien Cave, "Why Australia's COVID Death Rate Is Only One-Tenth of U.S. Level," *New York Times*, May 16, 2022, A1–6.
13. Kwame Anthony Appiah, *Cosmopolitanism: Ethics in a World of Strangers*, Norton, 2007.
14. Moderna press release, "Global Public Health Strategy," March 16, 2022.
15. Morgan Hines, and Andrea Mandell," *USA Today*, March 25, 2020, archived from the original published on March 27, 2020.
16. Michael Levenson, "Cruise Line Found at Fault for Hundreds Getting COVID," *New York Times*, October 27, 2023, A14.
17. "Biweekly Confirmed COVID Deaths," *Our World in Data*, https://ourworldindata.org/grapher/biweekly-covid-deaths?tab=chart&country=~USA (accessed March 29, 2024).

ACKNOWLEDGMENTS

Alfred Garwood, a retired librarian, philosopher, and entrepreneur, read every chapter carefully and made invaluable suggestions. He also sent me articles of interest, as did longtime former colleague Dennis Watts. Many physicians who worked though the worst of Covid talked to me, not all at UAB, but none wished to go on record, for reasons explained in chapter 4. I also benefited from presentations of premed students in my bioethics seminar, especially Joy Duan's on Long Covid. Rhonda Curry, a retired lawyer and administrative law judge and my former classmate at William & Mary, gave me insights into America's disability system.

Books Cited

Barr, William, *One Damn Thing after Another: Memoirs of an Attorney General*, William Morrow, 2022.

Barry, John, *The Great Influenza: The Story of the Deadliest Pandemic in History*, Viking, 2004.

Brix, Deborah, MD, *Silent Invasion*, HarperCollins, 2022.

Christakis, Nicholas, *Apollo's Arrow: The Profound and Enduring Impact of Coronavirus on the Way We Live*, Little, Brown, 2021.

COVID Crisis Group, *Lessons from the COVID War: An Investigative Report*, New York: Public Affairs Press, 2023.

Duffy, Bobby, *The Perils of Perception: Why We're Wrong about Nearly Everything*, London: Atlantic Books, 2019.

Fassin, Didier, and Marion Fourcade, *Pandemic Exposures: Economy and Society in the Time of the Coronavirus*, HAU Books, 2022, Society for Ethnographic Theory, www.haubooks.org.

Fauci, Anthony, *On Call: A Doctor's Journey in Public Service*, Viking, 2024.

Gandhi, Monica, *Endemic: A Post-Pandemic Playbook*, Mayo Clinic Press, 2023.

Gottlieb, Scott, MD, *Uncontrolled Spread*, HarperCollins, 2021.

Iyer, Ravi, MD, *The Reaper's Dance: 1000 Days of COVID*, Kindle Desktop Publishing, 3rd edition, 2023.

Kucharski, Adam, *The Rules of Contagion*, New York: Basic Books, 2020.

Kushner, Jared, *Breaking History: A White House Memoir*, Broadside Books, 2022.

Lewis, Michael, *The Premonition: A Pandemic Story*, Norton, 2021.

Loomis, Joshua, *Epidemics: The Impact of Germs and Their Power over Humanity*, New York: Prager, 2020.

Lowenstein, Fiona (ed.), *The Long COVID Survival Guide*, The Experiment, LLC, 2022.

MacKenzie, Deborah, *COVID-19: The Pandemic That Never Should Have Happened and How to Stop the Next One*, Hatchette, 2020.

McNeil, Donald, Jr. *The Wisdom of Plagues: Lessons from 25 Years of Covering Pandemics*, Simon & Schuster, 2024.

Meadows, Mark, *The Chief's Chief*, All Seasons Press, 2021.

Nocera, Joe, and Bethany McLean, *The Big Fail: What the Pandemic Revealed about Who America Protects and Who It Leaves Behind*, New York: Penguin, 2023.

Pence, Gregory, *Pandemic Bioethics*, Broadview Press, 2021.

Preston, Richard, *The Hot Zone: The Terrifying True Story of the Origins of the Ebola Virus*, Anchor Press, 1995.

Quammen, David, *Breathless: The Scientific Race to Defeat a Deadly Virus*, Simon & Schuster, 2022.

Trump, Mary, PhD, *The Reckoning: Our Nation's Trauma and Finding a Way to Heal*, St. Martin's, 2021.

Woodward, Bob, *Rage*, Simon & Schuster, 2020.

Wright, Lawrence, *The Plague Year: America in the Time of* COVID, Penguin Random House, 2023.

INDEX

About the Author

Philosopher Peter Singer called Gregory Pence's previous book on Covid an "extraordinary achievement," and this book takes that work one step further. Pence has taught at the medical center at the University of Alabama in Birmingham (UAB) for nearly fifty years, and he wrote the bestselling text *Medical Ethics* with McGraw-Hill, now in its tenth edition, as well as nine trade books with Rowman & Littlefield, including *Overcoming Addiction* and *Designer Food*, both *Choice* magazine Outstanding Academic Titles. He has published over seventy op-ed essays in periodicals such as the *Wall Street Journal*, the *New York Times*, the *Los Angeles Times*, *Newsweek*, the *Chronicle of Higher Education*, and the *Birmingham News*. He has won the three major teaching awards at UAB, and his ethics bowl teams have won four national championships. In 2001, he testified before a congressional committee on C-SPAN, speaking against a bill to make embryonic and reproductive cloning a federal crime. His fights against infectious diseases include being the chair of Birmingham AIDS Outreach's Board in the 1980s, and some of the ethical issues of that era reappeared with Covid, issues he discusses in this book.